Epilepsy in Resource Limited Settings

Focused on the understandings and impacts of epilepsy in resource-limited settings, particularly those in the Global South, this important book provides a thorough examination of how the condition can be managed to promote better quality of life.

This book is informed by global initiatives, including the Intersectoral Global Action Plan (IGAP) on epilepsy established by the World Health Organization in 2022. The first two chapters are centred on two broad but competing perspectives on epilepsy, the spiritual and the biological, which are followed by chapters covering the determinants and prevention of epilepsy, and first aid, guidance and counselling. This book moves on to outline the disadvantages, impacts and challenges of epilepsy, and initiatives to address the condition at regional and global levels, spotlighting responses in Africa, Asia and the Pacific, the Caribbean, the Middle East and North Africa, and Latin America. The final section of this book focuses on social management, individual resilience and social services, with a concluding chapter outlining a new Integrative Model for Managing Epilepsy (IMME).

Written by an author with extensive experience designing and leading epilepsy programmes both internationally and in sub-Saharan Africa, this book will interest Social Work, Public Health, Nursing, Medical, Counselling, Community Health scholars, students and practitioners.

Rugare Mugumbate is a Senior Lecturer in the School of Health & Society, Faculty of Arts, Humanities and Social Sciences, University of Wollongong, Australia. He is a Senior Research Associate in the Department of Social Work & Community Development, Faculty of Humanities, University of Johannesburg, South Africa. He is Chairperson of Social Work Taskforce, International League Against Epilepsy. He is a Researcher and Senior Social Worker in Epilepsy Resource Centre, Zimbabwe.

Epilepsy in Resource Limited Settings

Managing Quality of Life

Rugare Mugumbate

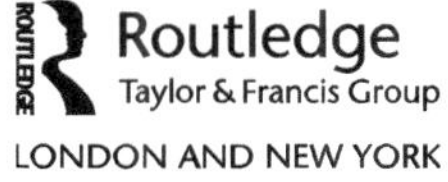

Routledge
Taylor & Francis Group

LONDON AND NEW YORK

First published 2025
by Routledge
4 Park Square, Milton Park, Abingdon, Oxon OX14 4RN

and by Routledge
605 Third Avenue, New York, NY 10158

Routledge is an imprint of the Taylor & Francis Group, an informa business

British Library Cataloguing-in-Publication Data
A catalogue record for this book is available from the British Library

ISBN: 978-1-032-80714-0 (hbk)
ISBN: 978-1-032-99194-8 (pbk)
ISBN: 978-1-003-60286-6 (ebk)

DOI: 10.4324/9781003602866

Typeset in Times New Roman
by codeMantra

Contents

Tables

Tools and models

Information boxes

Foreword

This book aims to bridge gaps in knowledge and government social support systems for those affected by epilepsy, particularly in resource-limited settings of the Global South. It brings together knowledge from social work, as well as various disciplines, drawing on experiences from different cultures and regions, while emphasising the importance of community and collaboration.

Epilepsy is often shrouded in stigma and misunderstanding, which can lead to significant disadvantages and barriers to care and support. This book shares research and examples of social management interventions and proposes a model to better manage epilepsy now and into the future. This knowledge empowers readers—whether they are students, professionals or advocates—to enhance the quality of life for those living with epilepsy.

This book explores the social, cultural and economic factors and other determinants that influence the lives of individuals with this condition. The integration of various perspectives supports a holistic approach to health and well-being, which considers the interconnectedness of physical, mental, spiritual and social health.

In my work for several years as a medical practitioner and founder of social services in my country, along with my contributions to global epilepsy organisations such as the International Bureau for Epilepsy (IBE) and the International League Against Epilepsy (ILAE), as well as my involvement in the Middle East and North Africa (MENA) region and the Africa region as President of the Epilepsy Alliance Africa (EAA), I have come to the conclusion that collaboration among people with epilepsy, medical and social professionals and caregivers is a stronger way forward.

As you read the chapters that follow, I encourage you to keep an open mind and reflect on how to consider how the knowledge presented can be applied in your own context. Together, we can contribute to a world where understanding and service replace disadvantage, fear and ignorance, ensuring that all individuals with epilepsy receive the empowering support and services they deserve.

Dr. Najib Kissani
Professor in Neurology
Former Head of Neurology Department, University Hospital Mohamed VI, Marrakech, Morocco
President of Moroccan League Against Epilepsy
Member of Telemedicine Commission in International League Against Epilepsy (ILAE)
Editor in Chief of the *African & Middle East Epilepsy Journal* (AMEEJ)

Preface

In the Global South, various initiatives have been implemented to improve the quality of life of people with epilepsy and their families. In Africa, Latin America, the Caribbean, Asia and the Pacific, and the Middle East and North Africa (MENA), governments, epilepsy associations and researchers have been active, working individually and together at local, national and regional levels. Each region has implemented programmes and has achievements to show. However, there are also challenges, such as healthcare access, cultural attitudes and resource availability. These difficulties are specific to each region, but there are common ones. Understanding these global trends, challenges and successful approaches will be useful for current and future programming.

Between 2002 and 2005, several declarations were made on epilepsy in all regions of the world, including Africa which is my region. Ten years later, in 2015, a global declaration on epilepsy was made, this time led by the World Health Organization (WHO) and global epilepsy and brain organisations. All the declarations had medical and social goals for reducing seizures and stigma. As a social worker, the social goals interested me more; however, it is important to note that medical and social goals complement each other. In my view, none can succeed without the other. This view is also supported by my experience, as a social worker for 15 years at two epilepsy organisations in Zimbabwe and is supported by my research on epilepsy, disability, employment and Indigenous knowledges (Mugumbate, 2010; Mugumbate & Nyanguru, 2013; Mugumbate & Mushonga, 2013; Mugumbate & Gray, 2016, 2017a, 2017b, 2021; Mugumbate, Riphagenn, & Gathara, 2017; Mugumbate & Zimba, 2018; Mugumbate et al., 2022, 2023).

My most extensive research on epilepsy was carried out in Zimbabwe between 2024 and 2017 as part of my doctoral programme on epilepsy, disability, employment and social justice at the University of Newcastle in Australia. Most chapters of this book contain information from this research.

My research has obviously motivated this book, but there are other motivations too. One is my policy contributions to epilepsy at the local (Zimbabwe), regional (Africa) and international levels. I have worked for and provided leadership to various epilepsy organisations and programmes, including in committees of the Africa Epilepsy Alliance (Secretary General, 2023–2025), International Bureau for Epilepsy (Vice President, 2017–2019) and the International League Against Epilepsy (Chair of the Social Work and Social Services Section, 2019–2025).

In 2018, I addressed the WHO General Assembly in Geneva, Switzerland during a session that involved the International Bureau for Epilepsy (IBE), International League Against Epilepsy (ILAE) and the International Brain Organisation (IBRO). My statement (Information box 0.1) called for accelerated action on epilepsy.

Information box 0.1 Statement during the WHO General Assembly

Statement read at the Seventy-First World Health Assembly (A71/1) 2018 calling for implementation of WHA68.20 Resolution on Epilepsy

Agenda Item: 20.3.2.3 F. Global burden of epilepsy and the need for co-ordinated action at the country level to address its health, social and public knowledge implications (resolution WHA68.20, 2015).

Statement by the International Bureau for Epilepsy (IBE)

Your Excellences, Honorable Ministers, Ambassadors, Delegates:

The International Bureau for Epilepsy envisions a world where understanding and care replace ignorance and fear of epilepsy. Epilepsy affects people of all ages and all ethnicities. Close to 80% of the 50 million people living with epilepsy live in low- and middle-income countries. It is unacceptable that 75% of people with epilepsy living in low- and middle-income countries do not have access to treatment. Approximately 65% of these individuals could be treated easily with inexpensive daily medication that costs as little as US$5 per year. Without access, these people will continue to live in poverty and be at risk. Worldwide the number of cases of unexpected death in epilepsy is estimated at 60,000 per year. In low- and middle-income countries, the mortality and morbidity rates are even higher because of status epilepticus and drowning. In every part of the world, people with epilepsy and their families suffer from human rights violations, stigma, social isolation, seizure-related injuries and discrimination. Persons with epilepsy have access barriers in schooling, employment and healthcare. WHO demonstration projects have indicated that it is possible to diagnose and treat most people with epilepsy at the primary healthcare level without the use of sophisticated equipment. To do this, we need to have a commitment from governments that epilepsy is a public health priority. Progress towards achieving the goals of WHA68.20 has been slow. On behalf of persons living with epilepsy and their care providers, we ask:

1 for a new report on the implementation of the resolution WHA 68.20 to be prepared and discussed again at the 74th World Health Assembly in 2021 and

2 for the development of a Global Action Plan on Epilepsy.

I thank you.

As a result of several years of global advocacy, the Intersectoral Global Action Plan (IGAP) on epilepsy was put in place by the WHO. The IGAP seeks to reduce the knowledge, policy and treatment gap in epilepsy, in order to improve the quality of life of people with epilepsy and their families (WHO, 2022, 2024). This book's key themes are motivated by the IGAP and the declarations on epilepsy. The themes are filling the quality of life, policy gap in epilepsy, and resource and income gaps in epilepsy.

This book targets human service students, professionals and researchers in the Global South but will be applicable to those in the Global North too. The objectives of this book are:

- Increase the understanding of, and interventions to improve the quality of life of people with epilepsy in resource-limited settings.
- Increase the understanding of, and interventions to reduce the income gap in epilepsy in resource-limited settings.
- Increase the understanding of, and interventions to reduce the policy gap in epilepsy in resource-limited settings.
- Enhancing the skills of those providing social interventions to improve the quality of life of people with epilepsy in epilepsy in resource-limited settings.

This book focuses on human and social services, whereas previous books have focused on health and medical services. Furthermore, this book focuses on resource-limited settings, mainly those of the Global South where, until now, there was no book that focuses on the social management of epilepsy.

Some chapters in this book are based on doctoral research supervised by Professors Mel Gray and Amanda Howard at the University of Newcastle. I am indebted to them.

References

Mugumbate, J., & Gray, M. (2016). Social justice and disability policy in Southern Africa. *Journal of Social Development in Africa, 31*(2), 7–24.

Mugumbate, J., & Gray, M. (2017a). Competing traditional and medical treatments of epilepsy in Harare, Zimbabwe. *African and Middle East Journal of Epilepsy, 6*(2), 1–9.

Mugumbate, J., & Gray, M. (2017b). Individual resilience as a strategy to counter employment barriers for people with epilepsy in Zimbabwe. *Epilepsy and Behaviour.* March, doi:10.1016/j.yebeh.2017.06.018

Mugumbate, J., & Gray, M. (2021). Employment rights for people with epilepsy in Zimbabwe: A social justice perspective. In V. Sewpaul, L. Kreitzer & T. Raniga (Eds.), *The tensions between culture and human rights. Emancipatory social work and Afrocentricity in a Global World,* (pp. 88–99). Calgary: University of Calgary Press.

Mugumbate, J., & Mushonga, J. (2013). Myths, perceptions, and incorrect knowledge surrounding epilepsy in rural Zimbabwe: A study of the villagers in Buhera District. *Epilepsy & Behavior, 27*(1), 144–147. doi:10.1016/j.yebeh.2012.12.036

Mugumbate, J., & Nyanguru, A. (2013). Measuring the challenges of people with epilepsy in Harare, Zimbabwe. *Neurology Asia, 18*(1), 29–33.

Mugumbate, J., Riphagenn, H., & Gathara, R. (2017). The role of social workers in the social management of epilepsy in Africa. In M. Gray (Ed.), *The handbook of social work and social development in Africa* (pp. 168–180). London: Routledge.

Mugumbate, J., & Zimba, A. (2018). Epilepsy in Africa: Past, present, and future. *Epilepsy & Behavior, 7*, 239–241. doi:10.1016/j.yebeh.2017.10.009

Mugumbate, J. R. (2010). *Global Campaign Against Epilepsy (GCAE) Zimbabwe Report.* Harare: Epilepsy Support Foundation.

Mugumbate, J. R., Kissani, N., Acevedo, K., Mugumbate, C., Janneh, A., Lilia Núñez-Orozco, L., Mauricio, O. A., & Ibrahim, E A. A. (2022). First Aid (FA) and First Guidance (FG) for epilepsy seizures: Key considerations and recommendations for developing regions of the world. *Journal of Social Issues in Non-Communicable Conditions & Disability, 1*(1), 11–24.

Mugumbate, R., Klevor, R., Aguirre, M. O., Massi, G.D., Yaqoob, N., Acevedo, K., Yewnetu, E., Kanyabutembo, C., Ibrahim, E.A.A., Boutadghart, S., Janneh, A., & Kissani, N. (2023). Epilepsy awareness days, weeks, and months: Their roles in the fight against epilepsy and the intersectoral global action plan on epilepsy and other neurological disorders. *Epilepsy & Behavior, 148*, 109457. doi:10.1016/j.yebeh.2023.109457

World Health Organization (WHO). (2022). Intersectoral global action plan on epilepsy and other neurological disorders 2022–2031. Retrieved November 3, 2022 from https://www.who.int/news/item/28-04-2022-draft-intersectoral-global-action-plan-on-epilepsy-and-other-neurological-disorders-2022-2031

World Health Organization (WHO). (2024). Epilepsy. Retrieved from https://www.who.int/news-room/fact-sheets/detail/epilepsy

Acronyms and abbreviations

AU	African Union
CEMM	Comprehensive epilepsy management model epilepsy
CPRD	Convention on the Rights of Persons with Disabilities
CT scan	Computed Tomography scan
DPM	Disabled People's Movement
DPO	Disabled Persons Organisations
EAA	Epilepsy Alliance Africa
EDLIZ	Essential Drugs List for Zimbabwe
EEG	Electroencephalography
ERCZ	Epilepsy Resource Centre Zimbabwe
ESA	Epilepsy South Africa
ESF	Epilepsy Support Foundation
FODPZ	Federation of Disabled Persons in Zimbabwe
GCAE	Global Campaign Against Epilepsy
IBE	International Bureau for Epilepsy
ICF	International Classification of Functioning, Disability and Health
IFSW	International Federation of Social Workers
ILAE	International League Against Epilepsy
ILO	International Labour Organisation
IMME	Integrative Model for Managing Epilepsy
MRI	Magnetic Resonance Imaging
NGO	Nongovernment Organisation
SADC	Southern Africa Development Community
SAFOD	Southern Africa Federation of the Disabled
SINTEF	Foundation for Scientific and Industrial Research at the Norwegian Institute of Technology
SDGs	Sustainable Development Goals
UN	United Nations
UNDP	United Nations Development Program
UPIAS	Union of the Physically Impaired Against Segregation
WHO	World Health Organization
ZINATHA	Zimbabwe National African Traditional Healers' Association
ZLAE	Zimbabwe League Against Epilepsy

1 Perspectives and approaches to epilepsy globally

Epilepsy is a condition characterised by the occurrence of recurring seizures, typically defined as two or more seizures. A seizure is an isolated event of epilepsy with symptoms that can include uncontrolled jerking of the body or one of its parts, stiffening of the body muscles and loss of consciousness. An episode is an instance of seizures, which can include one or more seizures in a short period of time. Not all seizures are epilepsy related, some may only happen once, and some may happen more than two times but temporarily. Epilepsy has been a subject of debate since time immemorial. The key debates are on causes, treatment, determinants and status of people with epilepsy in society. Viewed from another angle, these debates are about the medical, psychological, social, economic and spiritual aspects of epilepsy. This introductory chapter covers the key debates in epilepsy. Even though the book's focus is on resource-limited settings, this chapter's focus is global to reflect common understandings of the condition. This chapter starts with a discussion of epilepsy in everyday life, followed by key perspectives and models. At the end, the current understanding of epilepsy, based on modern scientific research, is summarised.

Epilepsy in everyday life

Living with epilepsy is largely defined by stigma of having a condition that families and communities do not want to be associated with because they think it is contagious, an indication of weakness in the genes of the family, a source of social disadvantages. This stigma leads to exclusion in society. However, for people with epilepsy this is a secondary problem, the primary problem is having unexpected uncontrolled seizures, especially in public, and often unconsciously. The key priorities for families, community and people with epilepsy are therefore shaped by these everyday experiences. Since time immemorial, the priority for society has been to find a cure for epilepsy, and this remains the top priority today because a cure has not been found. How to address this priority has evolved in all regions of the world, but there is now consensus that treatment with tested and verified medicines offers the best solution, even though there is no such a medicine for a significant number of epilepsies. To understand that there are several types of epilepsies, over 30 and the presentation of epilepsy will vary from person to person.

DOI: 10.4324/9781003602866-1

Many people with epilepsy stay at home most of the time because of fear of dangerous environments outside their home especially given that seizures are unpredictable. At home, there are also carers who are able to look after, provide first aid and guidance when needed. Because of these fears, socialisation, education and training opportunities are often limited, and this leads to reduction in income opportunities.

Epilepsy can make people more likely to get injured, experience disabilities, or even face life-threatening situations, including death. In resource-limited settings, access to medical care and support may be limited, making it even more difficult for individuals with epilepsy to manage their condition. When someone has a seizure, they might fall or hurt themselves, and serious seizures may require immediate medical attention. There is also a risk of sudden unexpected death in epilepsy (SUDEP). Living with epilepsy can bring extra risks and challenges, especially in areas where resources are scarce, affecting daily life and overall well-being.

The recurrence of seizure episodes varies. For other people, seizures may recur every hour, for others every day, week, month, season or year. The number of seizures per each episode varies. Others may have just one seizure, and others may have several repeatedly. An episode usually does not last five minutes, if it does, this becomes a medical emergency. Seizures are usually unpredictable for most people; however, some people may have warning signs.

Another key priority is to foster acceptance of people with epilepsy. This has proved to be a difficult task because the condition is thought to be contagious yet it is not at all. Associated with this belief, other people think all epilepsies can be inherited, which is not true. These understandings of epilepsy are related to what each community believes to be the causes and treatments of the condition. The proceeding sections provide more information about the understandings of epilepsy in different cultures.

The spiritual perspective

Spirituality mainly comes from culture of which religion is the main part of culture linked to it. There are many religions in the world, including African, Abrahamic which includes Judaism, Christianity and Islam, Asian which includes Hinduism and Buddhism, European, Caribbean and Pacific. Globally, religion sees epilepsy as a condition influenced by supernatural forces or spiritual causes (Baker, 2002; Ferguson, 2012; Mushi et al., 2011). Epilepsy is viewed as a contagious condition treatable through cultural or religious practices—sometimes termed complementary or alternative therapies—and not through conventional biomedical methods (Green, 2000). In many cultures, spiritual perspectives have proved incompatible wither cases dominate biomedical approaches (Mushi et al., 2011; Mutanana & Mutara, 2015; Quereshi et al., 2017; Winkler et al., 2009).

Epilepsy is seen to have supernatural causes, signalling divine blessing or punishment or demonic possession (Devinsky & Lai, 2008; Magiorkinis, Diamantis, Sidiropoulou, & Panteliadis, 2014). In Sweden and Norway, epilepsy was strange, mysterious and caused by 'hidden people inhabiting the woods and the mountains' (Tuft, Nakken, & Kverndokk, 2017, p. 104). Treatment involved extracting the blood of criminals or itinerants with epilepsy or passing them through a hole in the sand to transfer the disease into the ground. Divine intervention as a method of treatment has been reported in many parts of the globe, if not all including Uganda, Tanzania, Malawi, Morocco, South Africa and Zambia in Africa (Baskind & Birbeck, 2005a, 2005b; Birbeck, 2000; Duggan, 2013; Ferguson, 2012; Keikelame & Swartz, 2015; Mushi et al., 2011; Winkler et al., 2009). In most of these countries, epilepsy was linked to witchcraft, curable only by traditional healers. In Malawi and South Africa, traditional healers claimed to treat the spiritual cause of epilepsy but agreed some types of epilepsy required medical treatment (Keikelame & Swartz, 2015). Green (2000) found many people with epilepsy in the Global South spent time and resources on traditional remedies, since they considered the 'treatment of seizures … the domain of traditional healers' (p. 805).

Due to fear of contagion, people with epilepsy used to be ostracised from the community and tied to trees in the forest, or, as in Zimbabwe, chained to posts or committed to mental institutions, or, in communities where epilepsy was viewed as a curse, people with epilepsy were killed (Epilepsy Support Foundation [ESF], 1992). This situation existed in most parts of the world (Baskind & Birbeck, 2005a; Ndoye et al., 2005). For example, in the USA, owners of public spaces had the right to deny people with epilepsy access until the 1970s, and 1971 in the United Kingdom (UK) (World Health Organisation [WHO], 2016). In India, China and many other countries, epilepsy provided grounds to annul a marriage (WHO, 2016). In other parts of the world, people with epilepsy were prevented from having children, while companies refused to hire people with epilepsy (WHO, 2016).

In Morocco, which has a majority Muslim population, epilepsy was a religious, supernatural and cultural condition caused by evil spirits or demons called *jinn* (Ferguson, 2012). Jinn was reported in other Muslim countries, such as the Kingdom of Saudi Arabia (Almutairi et al., 2016) and Afghanistan (Daber-Taleh, Uwe, & Rösche, 2017). A *fquih* or an imam, a religious scholar well versed in the Quran, used his supernatural powers to speak with, and expel, the jinn, while touching the patient. If this does not work, the *fquih* recites passages from the Quran or treated the 'possessed person' with smoke and scents. Sick people often wore charms and amulets with Quran verses on them to stave off evil. If none of these rituals worked, this meant the *jinn* had married the patient, parented children and was unwilling to leave. To prevent evil possession, people had to have faith in Allah and the Prophet Mohamed, pray and perform daily rituals and ablutions, and avoid haunted places, such as dark spaces and abandoned buildings (Ferguson, 2012) Witches, or *jadu/ dua*, are considered a possible cause of epilepsy in Afghanistan's traditional shamanist belief system (Daber-Taleh et al., 2017). Besides imams, magicians called *jadugar* treat epilepsy in Afghanistan though medical treatment is also condoned (Daber-Taleh et al., 2017). Resultantly, as in traditional African societies, the treatment of epilepsy in Islamic societies combines medical and spiritual methods (Almutairi et al., 2016; Daber-Taleh et al., 2017; Ferguson, 2012).

The biological perspective

Also referred to as the physical approach, the biological perspective argues that epilepsy is caused by malfunctioning components of the human body. The treatment focuses on correcting or mitigating the part of the body that is malfunctioning. The approaches to treatment vary, but often complement each other. There are four approaches, herbal, dietary, surgical and electro-pharmacological which is the most popular and most successful to date. The herbal approach uses herbs derived from plants, animals, soil, water or human body to treat epilepsy. Herbs can be liquids or solids, or mixtures. They can be ingested via the mouth, breathed in or bathed in water. The dietary approach can be seen as part of the herbal; however, the focus is on the food that a person consumes. The ketogenic diet, which controls energy that goes to the brain, is an example of a dietary approach. A ketogenic diet is high in fats and low in carbohydrates. Other types of epilepsy result from a tumour or wound in the brain which can be removed surgically. The electro-pharmacological approach is based on the electrical theory of epilepsy founded in the 1850s by Hitzig and Todd (Magiorkinis et al., 2014). Though herbal treatment continued, Sir Locock discovered the usefulness of potassium bromide in the treatment of epilepsy in 1857, which remained popular until the discovery of phenobarbital in 1912 (Magiorkinis et al., 2014). The electrical theory of epilepsy and the classification of epilepsy into idiopathic or sympathetic and petit or grand mal seizures became widely accepted (Magiorkinis et al., 2014).

In the 1930s, Hans Berger proved that epilepsy arose from electrical activity in the brain and used that information to invent electroencephalography (EEG), followed by the discovery of the first drugs for the treatment of epilepsy around 1940, though these early medicines had many side effects (Ferguson, 2012). Ongoing pharmacological research resulted in the effective and affordable medicines used today. Several methods of treatment for severe epilepsy developed, including surgery, though medication remained the primary treatment for more than 70% of epilepsy cases (Ferguson, 2012). Despite advances in medicine, including diagnostic and surgical equipment, there was still no complete cure for seizures, with most people with epilepsy remaining on life-long, daily medication to control their seizures. Medicines are often classified as first-, second- or third-line, with the latter being most effective but expensive (WHO, 2016). Even if fully treated, some people with epilepsy were susceptible to seizures triggered by, *inter alia*, fatigue, light, heat, hormonal changes due to pregnancy, menstruation or aging and lack of sleep or food (Dekker, 2002). Moreover, even with the advent and development of antiepileptic medication, several communities continued to rely on herbal remedies and spiritual healing, while prejudice against people with epilepsy remained in most countries (Ferguson, 2012).

Indigenous health theory

Indigenous health theory uses spiritual and biological understandings and is documented by the WHO. Terms such complementary, alternative, or non-conventional health are often associated with Indigenous health. These include the methods already discussed and many other ones including acupuncture which is popular in China and Ayurveda from India which combines *panchakarma* (five actions), yoga, massage, acupuncture and herbs to achieve holistic treatment. Other treatment approaches include a ketogenic diet and vagus-nerve and deep-brain or trigeminal nerve stimulation (International Bureau for Epilepsy [IBE], 2014).

Information box 1.1   Indigenous health theory

This theory is about valuing Indigenous methods of healing, health and well-being. The WHO defines Indigenous health or 'traditional health' as

> the sum total of knowledge, skills and practices based on the theories, beliefs and experiences indigenous to different cultures, whether explicable or not, that are used to maintain health, as well as to prevent, diagnose, improve or treat physical and mental illnesses.

Indigenous health values connection to land or environment, culture, spirituality, ancestry, family and community. Over 70%–80% of Africans use Indigenous health for most of their health needs. Allopathic medicine refers to the most dominant form of medicine today that is a system dominated by medical doctors, pharmacists, therapists and nurses who treat symptoms and diseases using drugs, radiation, surgery and other methods—also called bio-, conventional or orthodox. Key aspects of Indigenous health include the following:

1　It involves Indigenous methods from the people and was developed over many years. These methods are continuously evolving and new methods come every day.
2　Just like modern science-based medicine, Indigenous health methods have side effects, but their side effects are less severe.
3　The devaluing of Indigenous medicine is largely for economic reasons. Innovations of the Global North try to keep those of the Global South out of competition. There is competition for pharmacies, clinics, labs, patents, jobs, education, marketing, distribution and equipment.
4　When white people colonised Africa, they put in place laws to prohibit use and growth of Indigenous health. In Zimbabwe, South Africa, Zimbabwe, Zambia, Malawi, Namibia and other countries, they put in place Witchcraft Suppression Act (laws) and prohibited use and practice of Indigenous health.
5　The religion of Abraham with its three major sub-religions of Judaism, Christianity and Islam contributed significantly to devaluing and banning of Indigenous health as part of the large religious colonisation of Africa.

6 Indigenous medicine is capable of growth and improvement, but it faces several barriers including limited or no research funding, not included in school or university curriculum and stigmatisation.

7 Each type of medicine can be an alternative or complementary approach to the other; for example, modern science-based medicine can be alternative or complementary to Indigenous medicine and vice versa.

8 Both scientific and Indigenous knowledge can be the basis of each other's improvement. Most modern knowledge was based on Indigenous knowledges. Actually, there is a very thin line between scientific and Indigenous methods.

9 There has been theft of Indigenous knowledges and plants, and they end up being commercialised.

10 Modern medicine is based on trial and error and can be very unethical at times. Modern science has several scandals, and other parts of society have lost confidence in it. There are several conditions science has failed to explain and to treat.

11 There is a huge economic cost of neglecting Indigenous health methods. Universal health coverage cannot be achieved without Indigenous medicines.

12 Indigenous health is holistic not narrow. It focusses on the physical, psychological, social, spiritual, cultural, biological and environmental aspects of health.

13 It is natural not artificial.

14 It takes a bottom-up not top-down approach to health.

15 Sociocultural acceptance of Indigenous systems is high.

16 Drug dependence and overprescription are major issues with modern medicine.

Reproduced with permission from Africa Social Work and Development Network (ASWDNet) (2021)

In many countries, there are centres, departments or programmes dedicated to promoting various types of therapy. In 1978, at the Alma Ata conference, the WHO recommended that Indigenous health practices, including traditional birth attendance, should be integrated into national health systems. For instance, the WHO has established the Global Centre for Traditional Medicine (GCTM) in India, supported by a $250 million grant from the Government of India. Chinese Medicine is a major industry, and the African Union observes African Traditional Medicine Day each year on 31 August. The WHO African Region has guidelines for the registration of traditional medicines (TMs) in the region, and the period from 2001 to 2010 was designated as the Decade for African Traditional Medicine. South Africa has a National Reference Centre for African Traditional Medicines (NRCATM), the Traditional Health Practitioners Act (THPA) No. 22 of 2007 and a Directorate of Traditional Medicine (DTM) (ASWDNet, 2021). The WHO Congress on Traditional Medicine took place in Beijing, China, in 2008. It declared that governments have a duty to safeguard the health of their populations and should create national policies, regulations and standards to ensure the safe, appropriate and effective use of TM. The Congress also emphasised that TM should be advanced through research and innovation. The current WHO Traditional Medicine Strategy for 2014–2023 aims to harness TM's potential contribution to health, wellness and people-centred care. Its goals include promoting the safe and effective use of TM by regulating, researching and integrating TM products, practitioners and practices into health systems where suitable, as well as providing education and training for TM and complementary and alternative medicine (CAM) practitioners.

A modern scientific understanding of epilepsy

Modern science says seizures emanate from neurons in the brain, the nerve cells responsible for communication between the brain and the body, through the transmission of electrical impulses (Shorvon, 2009, 2024). A disturbance in this transmission process may result in an excessive discharge of 'messages' with body parts 'failing to take orders'. This may lead to lapses in attention, loss of sensation, jerking movements, falling or muscle stiffening. Such disturbances are largely the result of brain damage, either before or after birth (WHO, 2024). There are numerous causes of brain damage, including a lack of oxygen to the brain, head trauma at birth or due to accidents, substance—drug or alcohol—human violence, brain tumours, infections, such as meningitis and genetic syndromes. Most of these causes are preventable.

Seizures are classified as focal, generalised or of unknown origin (Fisher et al., 2017). Focal seizures, previously termed partial seizures, start from a localised part of the brain and they usually affect a small part of the body, while generalised seizures are widespread throughout the brain and, therefore, usually affect the whole body (Fisher et al., 2017). As the name suggests, unknown origin denotes inability to diagnose the cause of seizure onset. Seizures are characterised by stiffening body muscles (tonic), or not (atonic), jerky movements (clonic) or a combination of these (tonic-clonic) (Kiriakopoulos & Shafer, 2017). Some seizures involve loss of consciousness (Fisher et al., 2017). Seizures usually last one to three minutes. Those exceeding five minutes are treated as medical emergencies (Kiriakopoulos & Shafer, 2017; Shorvon, 2009). Following a seizure, a person may become confused, drowsy or depressed (Kiriakopoulos & Shafer, 2017). Some seizures are accompanied by groaning, jerking, cries, sudden falling, biting of the tongue, urinating or other acts that are often unpleasant to experience or witness (Kiriakopoulos & Shafer, 2017). The most recent classification of seizures was provided by the ILAE (Fisher et al. 2017). There are four classes: focal onset, generalised onset, unknown onset and unclassified. The characteristics of classes 1–3 are as follows:

1 Focal onset

- Aware
- Impaired awareness

  - Motor onset
  - Non-motor onset
  - Focal to bilateral tonic-clonic

2 Generalised onset

  - Motor
  - Non-motor (absence)

3 Unknown onset

  - Motor
  - Non-motor

4 Unclassified

Epilepsy requires life-long treatment with daily doses of antiepileptic medication or, in some cases, brain surgery. Uncontrolled epilepsy temporarily or permanently limits daily activities, such as speech, mobility, memory, sensation and social interaction (Birbeck & Kalichi, 2003). Control of epilepsy seizures has improved with advances in medicine that has significantly increased the number of people with epilepsy living seizure-free, productive lives (WHO, 2022). Shorvon (2009) reported that, with medical treatment, 60% had been found to be seizure-free within five years and 50% would have their epilepsy fully controlled to an extent that they could cease their antiepileptic medication; only about 30% of people with epilepsy in the Global North required regular medical attention, while 65% required occasional attention. Though the effectiveness of medical treatment is well established, research showed that 30% of people with epilepsy lacked effective treatment (Ferguson, 2012). Despite affordable treatment for epilepsy, most people with the condition in resource-poor settings were not properly diagnosed or treated (Baskind & Birbeck, 2005a; Shorvon, 2009).

Epilepsy is a chronic, non-communicable brain condition characterised by recurrent seizures and long-term stigma. It affects people of all ages. Approximately 50 million people worldwide are living with epilepsy, making it one of the most common neurological disorders. Nearly 80% of those affected reside in low- and middle-income countries, where access to appropriate treatment is often limited (WHO, 2022). The WHO estimates that up to 70% of individuals with epilepsy could potentially live seizure-free if they receive proper diagnosis and treatment. However, the risk of premature death among people with epilepsy can be up to three times higher than that of the general population. Worryingly, about 75% of individuals with epilepsy in low-income countries do not receive the treatment they need. Moreover, many people with epilepsy and their families face stigma and discrimination in various parts of the world, further complicating their lives. Addressing these challenges is essential for improving the well-being of those affected by this condition (WHO, 2024).

The outstanding question about epilepsy, which the spiritual and biological perspectives have not been able to answer, is that of cure. Epilepsy remains an incurable condition in spite of promises from both the spiritual and biological sides (WHO, 2022, 2024). If found, a cure would remove recurring seizures altogether. There are efforts to find a cure from all corners of the globe, and people with epilepsy, carers and those treating them are all anticipating a cure.

Information box 1.2   The major differences between spiritual (S) and biological (B) perspectives on epilepsy

Where does epilepsy come from?

S: It is spiritual, comes from supernatural holy or evil beings or deities.
B: *It is biological, it develops in the body.*

In the physical body, where does epilepsy reside?

S: *In the stomach or whole body or resides outside.*
B: *In the brain system.*

How is it treated?

S: *By removing the evil spirit (spiritually or herbally).*
B: *Herbally, dietary, surgically or pharmacologically.*

Cure?

S: *It can be cured.*
B: *There is no cure.*

What could be the role of the individual in the starting of epilepsy?

S: *The individual or their community member may be sinful or unjust.*
B: *The individual's brain is exposed to harmful substances, injury or infections, even before birth.*

How to prevent it?

S: *Live a life free of sin or injustice.*
B: *Protect the brain from harmful substances, injury or infections, for example.*

These different perspectives have shaped approaches to epilepsy; however, as indicated before, they at times all influence approaches. In the following section, different approaches to epilepsy will be discussed.

Approaches to epilepsy

The models for managing epilepsy include the medical, psychosocial, social, human rights, affirmative and economic.

Biomedical approach

This approach is also referred to as the pharmacological approach. Medically, epilepsy is a biological condition resulting from temporary or permanent impairments of the brain or its components that can be corrected with antiepileptic medication or surgery (WHO, 2022, 2024). The discovery of potassium bromide in 1857 strengthened the medical model (Scott, 1992). Supported by scientific research, medical treatment became the most effective method of seizure control globally. Internationally, medical progress has advanced the treatment of epilepsy through the Global Campaign Against Epilepsy (de Boer, 2010; de Boer, Engel Jr., & Prilipko, 2005; International League Against Epilepsy [ILAE], World Health Organisation [WHO], & International Bureau for Epilepsy [IBE], 2000). A study of resource-limited countries found that the cost was US$25 per person per year (Birbeck et al., 2012). This included the cost of training healthcare workers, first-line medicines and related costs. The cost of epilepsy medicines was lower than that for other chronic conditions (Birbeck et al., 2012). In India, Megiddo et al. (2016) estimated that US$5 was required to provide essential epilepsy medicines per person per year. However, this low cost has not resulted in increased government support for epilepsy (Birbeck et al., 2012; Kvalsund & Birbeck, 2012). In fact, the treatment gap in poor countries remains very high. As yet, antiepileptic medicines have not been made adequately available and affordable in developing countries and treatment facilities are overstretched and under resourced (Adamolekun & Meinardi, 1990; Baskind & Birbeck, 2005a; Meinardi, Scott, Reis, & Sander, 2001). The cost for medical management of epilepsy can be very low (WHO, 2024).

Psychosocial approach

While the medical model made strides in seizure control, it failed to address the structural conditions relegating people with epilepsy to the lowest rungs of society (Baskind & Birbeck, 2005a, 2005b; de Boer, 2010; Newton & Garcia, 2012; Shorvon, 2009). It has failed to deal with psychological aspects of epilepsy that include depression, anxiety, stigma and low self-esteem (Baker, 2002; Dekker, 2002) and social issues that include stigma, exclusion and disadvantage. Psychosocial interventions recognise the need for social measures—social policy, social services, social care and social support—for people with epilepsy. Most importantly, it recognises the structural factors that result in stigma, discrimination, marginalisation and exclusion of people with epilepsy (Dekker, 2002; Mugumbate, Riphagenn, & Gathara, 2017) and seeks to address the sociocultural, economic and political barriers to their participation in society, including unfriendly workplace policies and practices and ignorance about epilepsy. It highlights the importance of public education and awareness to reduce the stigma that is sometimes more difficult to overcome than the seizures (Dekker, 2002; Elger & Schmidt, 2008; Mugumbate et al., 2017). The psychosocial model has been promoted by the WHO in the International Classification of Functioning, Disability and Health framework. The International League Against Epilepsy (ILAE) and International Bureau for Epilepsy (IBE) have expanded the biopsychosocial model through their UN consultative status and affiliates in more than 100 countries (de Boer, 2010). The ILAE was formed in 1909 to advance prevention, diagnosis and treatment of epilepsy (ILAE et al., 2000). The IBE (2014) was formed in 1961 to ensure recognition of epilepsy in health and research and the protection of the rights of people with epilepsy. Together with the WHO, these two organisations embarked on the Global Campaign Against Epilepsy. They introduced International Epilepsy Day in 2015 and the WHO (2015) Resolution on Epilepsy to strengthen global care for epilepsy and advance the rights of people with epilepsy. Delegates at the World Health Assembly endorsed the Resolution on the Global Burden of Epilepsy and urged member states to strengthen their ongoing efforts to provide healthcare for people with epilepsy (WHO, 2015). They advocated the adoption, funding and implementation of policies, legislation and national healthcare plans of action for epilepsy management; integration of epilepsy prevention and management into primary healthcare; establishment of research centres and training programmes for non-specialist healthcare providers; capacity building for people with epilepsy and their carers; improved access to and affordability of antiepileptic medicines; public education to reduce misconceptions about epilepsy; timely treatment; improved access to education and employment; collaborations with civil society and other partners; and awareness raising to reduce stigma and discrimination (de Boer, 2010; Dekker, 2002; Elger & Schmidt, 2008).

Social approach

The social approach emphasises society's role in advancing human rights, equality of opportunity, non-discrimination, skills development, employment access and social protection for persons with disabilities. The social model of disability emerged from the ideas and principles of the Union of the Physically Impaired Against Segregation (UPIAS), an early disability rights organisation in the UK which promoted the idea that disability was more than an individual or personal issue (Oliver, 1990, 2009, 2013). It required social and political measures to ensure people with disabilities enjoyed the same opportunities as those in the general population (Morgan, 2012; Oliver, 2013). The Disabled Peoples Movement (DPM) promoted the social model of disability and a service-user perspective (Oliver, 2013). The social model highlighted the structural barriers and social inequalities endured by disabled people, who were among the poorest, most excluded, and devalued in society (Mtetwa, 2011, 2016; Oliver, 2013). It drew attention to stigma and discrimination caused by alienating or non-inclusive social structures, policies, processes and practices (Morgan, 2012; Oliver, 2009).

Human rights approach

At times called the advocacy approach, the human rights approach contends that other approaches focus on needs and deficits rather than entitlements and rights. The CRPD (United Nations [UN], 2006a) recognised disabled people's right to be treated with dignity and respect (Eide, 2012; Murungi, Mandlate, & Armah, 2013). Though they experienced life differently due to their disability, they were people (rather than disability) first and were entitled to the rights enjoyed by others in society (UN, 2006a). The human rights model gave rise to an empowering approach, in which people participated in decisions about their lives. It championed the enforceability of rights and called for social action and justice (Mgonela, 2010; Mtetwa, 2016; Murimi, 2013). Banks and Polack (2015) argued that rights and justice were intertwined. Fulfilment of rights meant enabling people to exercise choice, participate in society as peers, and access its opportunities and benefits (Fraser, 2008). It meant targeted programmes and mainstreaming disability for people to reach their full potential (Banks & Polack, 2015; Mgonela, 2010; Mtetwa, 2016; Murimi, 2013; Peta, McKenzie, & Kathard, 2015; UN, 2006b). The CRPD is a key pillar of the human rights approach because it mainstreamed disability in international development (Kett, Lang, & Trani, 2009; Visagie, Scheffler, & Schneider, 2013). However, Lang (2009) warned that the policy 'was not a sufficient instrument for the enforcement of disability rights and should not be perceived as a panacea that will end disability discrimination' (p. 1). Citing examples from Zimbabwe and Nigeria, Lang (2009) showed that local laws were difficult to change and politicians and the disability movement had conflicting goals.

Affirmation approach

The affirmative model is a non-tragic view of epilepsy that sees conditions the condition as part of human diversity. The model helps people with disability to take a positive view of their condition and helps society to see disability from the perspective of people with the condition. Its proponents contended that every human was impaired in some way though the degree of disability emanating from the impairment varied greatly (Lang, 2001; Swain & French, 2000). They called for people experiencing disability to celebrate and take pride in their unique identity and life-enriching attributes (McCormack & Collins, 2012). It was an extension of the social model of disability (Swain & French, 2000). However, the model has been criticised for neglecting the differences between disabled and able-bodied people. This could weaken the disability movement, especially if people with disabilities did not identify with the movement (Lang, 2001).

Economic approach

Income would help people with epilepsy acquire treatment services that they require. Income comes from family, work, employment, public welfare and non-public welfare. In the absence of employment, support from their governments would be expected to assist them. Given the low cost of epilepsy management, even resource-poor countries could provide free or affordable treatment for people with epilepsy (Chisholm, 2005; Megiddo et al., 2016). The WHO (2016) estimated that the cost of epilepsy treatment could be as low as US$5 per person per year. Megiddo et al. (2016) reported that 'expanding and publicly financing epilepsy treatment in India averts substantial disease burden' (p. 464). However, unemployment and the failure of most countries in the Global South to provide even the most basic first-line treatment resulted in significant economic and social impacts for people with epilepsy, their families, communities and nations. Employment and income perspectives are limited in epilepsy management, as in disability in general. However, Epilepsy South Africa (ESA, 2014) runs economic empowerment programmes, including sheltered workshops, and a mainstream employment programme named Epilepsy Disability Employment Support Services (eDESS). Sheltered workshops in Cape Town employ people with epilepsy in a factory that makes furniture for local and foreign markets and another producing mats and baskets. The eDESS links people with epilepsy, ESA and employers. Its major focus is employment preparation, to facilitate workplace adjustment and legal compliance, and supportive employment services, including skills development, short-term employment, induction and mentoring (ESA, 2014). The Employment Equity Act (Government of South Africa, 1998) promotes affirmative action, education and vocational training, and sensitisation of employers to foster positive attitudes towards people with epilepsy. Though the ESF in Zimbabwe does not run sheltered workshops, it promotes small self-help projects for its members and employer sensitisation initiatives. Self-help projects have been supported by the IBE in countries like Zambia, Kenya, Cameroon and Uganda.

Carers approach

The carers approach says that supporting individuals with epilepsy is crucial for their safety and well-being. Carers provide essential help by managing medications, offering emotional support, and ensuring a safe environment during seizures. They also educate others about epilepsy and advocate for the needs of those they care for, working alongside healthcare professionals to improve the overall quality of life for individuals living with the condition. The Epilepsy Alliance Africa (EAA) supports this approach, which is family-oriented and aligns well with the philosophy of Ubuntu in Africa. In 2024, the theme for EAA was 'Empowering Caregivers: A Journey of Giving, Receiving, and Valuing Care' (Epilepsy Alliance Africa [EAA], 2024). This approach is especially important in resource-limited settings, such as parts of sub-Saharan Africa, South Asia and some regions in Latin America, where access to healthcare may be restricted. In these areas, carers often become the primary support system for individuals with epilepsy, helping to fill gaps in care and fostering a supportive community network. By educating others about epilepsy, they reduce stigma and improve understanding, which is vital in regions where misinformation can be widespread. The carer approach enhances the quality of life for individuals with epilepsy and addresses the challenges faced in these environments.

Conclusion

From the previous discussion, it is clear that various factors affect epilepsy, including religious, cultural, social, environmental, psychological, genetic and political influences. These factors shape how people understand epilepsy and how individuals with epilepsy are treated in society. While there are some shared views on these influences, there are also ongoing debates about their roles. In resource-poor settings, such as many parts of the Global South, these factors can have a significant impact on the experience of epilepsy. Limited access to healthcare, education and support can make epilepsy a more challenging condition to manage. This chapter has explored the causes, symptoms and prevalence of epilepsy, and examined different perspectives on understanding and managing the condition. It has also highlighted how the social aspects of epilepsy can make it a disabling condition, especially in areas with fewer resources. The next chapter will explore two competing perspectives on the treatment of epilepsy—spiritual and biological and will expand on the ideas presented in this first chapter.

References

Adamolekun, B., & Meinardi, H. (1990). Problems of drug therapy of epilepsy in developing countries. *Tropical and Geographical Medicine, 42*(2), 178–181.

Africa Social Work and Development Network (ASWDNet). (2021). *Indigenous health theory*. Harare: ASWDNet.

Almutairi, M. A., Ansari, T., Sami, W., & Baz, S. (2016). Public knowledge and attitudes toward epilepsy in Majmaah. *Journal of Neurosciences in Rural Practice, 7*(4), 499–503. doi:10.4103/0976-3147.188622

Banks, L. M., & Polack, S. (2015). The economic costs of exclusion and gains of inclusion of people with disabilities. Evidence from low and middle income countries. Retrieved January 13, 2016 from https://disabilitycentre.lshtm.ac.uk/files/2014/07/Costs-of-Exclusion-and-Gains-of-Inclusion-Report.pdf

Baskind, R., & Birbeck, G. L. (2005a). Epilepsy care in Zambia: A study of traditional healers. *Epilepsia, 46*(7), 1121–1126. doi:10.1111/j.1528-1167.2005.03505.x

Baskind, R., & Birbeck, G. L. (2005b). Epilepsy-associated stigma in sub-Saharan Africa: The social landscape of a disease. *Epilepsy & Behavior, 7*(1), 68–73. doi:10.1016/j.yebeh.2005.04.009

Birbeck, G. L. (2000). Seizures in rural Zambia. *Epilepsia, 41*(3), 277–281.

Birbeck, G. L., Chomba, E., Mbewe, E., Atadzhanov, M., Haworth, A., & Kansembe, H. (2012). The cost of implementing a nationwide program to decrease the epilepsy treatment gap in a high gap country. *Neurology International, 4*(3), e14. doi:10.4081/ni.2012.e14

Birbeck, G. L., & Kalichi, E. M. N. (2003). The functional status of people with epilepsy in rural Sub-Saharan Africa. *Journal of the Neurological Sciences, 209*(1/2), 65. doi:10.1016/S0022-510X(02)00467-7

Chisholm, D. (2005). Cost-effectiveness of first-line drug treatments in the developing world: A population-level analysis. *Epilepsia, 46*, 751–559.

Daber-Taleh, S., Uwe, W., & Rösche, J. (2017). Knowledge and attitude towards epilepsy among students of economics in Herat, Afghanistan. *Neurology Asia, 22*(1), 1–8.

de Boer, H. M. (2010). Epilepsy stigma: Moving from a global problem to global solutions. *Seizure, 19*(10), 630–636. doi:10.1016/j.seizure.2010.10.017

de Boer, H., Engel Jr., J., & Prilipko, L. (2005). Global campaign against epilepsy. *Atlas Epilepsy Care in the World*, 82–83.

Dekker, P. A. (2002). *Epilepsy a manual for medical and clinical officers in Africa* (Revised ed.). Geneva: WHO.

2013). Epilepsy and its effects on children and families in rural Uganda. *African Health Sciences, 13*(3), 613–623. doi:10.4314/ahs.v13i3.14

Eide, A. H. (2012). *Education, employment and barriers for young people with disabilities in Southern Africa*. Paris: UNESCO.

Elger, C. E., & Schmidt, D. (2008). Modern management of epilepsy: A practical approach. *Epilepsy & Behavior, 12*(4), 501–539. doi:10.1016/j.yebeh.2008.01.C03

Epilepsy Alliance Africa (EAA) (2024). Epilepsy stripes week. Retrieved from https://epilepsyalliance.africasocialwork.net/stripes-week/

Epilepsy South Africa (ESA). (2014). eDESS (Epilepsy Disability Employment Support Services). Western Cape: Epilepsy South Africa.

Epilepsy Support Foundation (ESF). (1992). *Pfari muZimbabwe/Epilepsy in Zimbabwe*. Documentary. Harare: ESF.

Ferguson, C. (2012). Perceptions of epilepsy in Morocco seen by an American Neuroscientist. *North African and Middle East Epilepsy Journal, 1*(4), 4–7.

Fisher, R. S., Cross, J. H., French, J. A., Higurashi, N., Hirsch, E., Jansen, F. E., & Zuberi, S. M. (2017). Operational classification of seizure types by the International League against Epilepsy. Retrieved February 13, 2017 from https://www.ilae.org/visitors/centre/documents/ClassificationSeizureILAE-2016.pdf

Fraser, N. (2008). *Scales of justice. Reimaging political space in a globalizing world*. Cambridge: Polity Press.

Government of South Africa. (1998). *Employment Equity Act*. Cape Town: Government of South Africa.

Green, C. E. (2000) *Indigenous theory of contagious disease*. Lanham, MD: Altamira.

International Bureau for Epilepsy (IBE). (2014). *What is epilepsy?* Retrieved December 12, 2016 from https://www.ibe-epilepsy.org/what-is-epilepsy-2/

International League against Epilepsy (ILAE), World Health Organisation (WHO), & International Bureau for Epilepsy (IBE). (2000). *African declaration on epilepsy*. Retrieved July 12, 2015 from https://www.who.int/mental_health/neurology/epilepsy/african_declaration_2000.pdf

Keikelame, M. J., & Swartz, L. (2015). 'A thing full of stories': Traditional healers' explanations of epilepsy and perspectives on collaboration with biomedical health care in Cape Town. *Transcultural Psychiatry, 52*(5), 659–680. doi:10.1177/1363461515571626

Kett, M., Lang, R., & Trani, J.-F. (2009). Disability, development and the dawning of a new convention: A cause for optimism? *Journal of International Development, 21*(5), 649–661. doi:10.1002/jid.1596

Kiriakopoulos, E., & Shafer, P. O. (2017). 2017 Revised classification of seizures. Retrieved June 14, 2017 from https://www.epilepsy.com/learn/types-seizures/tonic-clonic-seizures

Kvalsund, M. P., & Birbeck, G. L. (2012). Epilepsy care challenges in developing countries. *Current Opinion in Neurology, 25*(2), 179–186. doi:10.1097/WCO.0b013e328350baf8

Lang, R. (2001). *The development and critique of the social model of disability*. London: Leonard Cheshire Disability and Inclusive Development Centre.

Lang, R. (2009). The United Nations Convention on the right and dignities for persons with disability: A panacea for ending disability discrimination? *ALTER – European Journal of Disability Research / Revue Européenne de Recherche sur le Handicap, 3*(3), 266–285. doi:10.1016/j.alter.2009.04.001

Madzokere, C. (1997). Life experiences of people with epilepsy. A study of Highfield high density residential area in Harare, Zimbabwe. *EPICADEC News (biannual newsletter of Foundation Epilepsy Care Developing Countries), 10*(97), 19–21.

Magiorkinis, E., Diamantis, A., Sidiropoulou, K., & Panteliadis, C. (2014). Highlights in the history of epilepsy: The last 200 years. *Epilepsy Research and Treatment, 582039,* 1–13.

McCormack, C., & Collins, B. (2012). The Affirmative Model of disability: A means to include disability orientation in Occupational Therapy? *British Journal of Occupational Therapy, 75*(3), 156–158. doi:10.4276/030802212X13311219571909

Megiddo, I., Colson, A, Chisholm, D., Dua, T., Nandi, A., & Laxminarayan, R. (2016) Health and economic benefits of public financing of epilepsy treatment in India: An agent-based simulation model. *Epilepsia, 57*(3), 464–474. doi:10.1111/epi.13294

Meinardi, H., Scott, R. A., Reis, R., & Sander, J. W. (2001). The treatment gap in epilepsy: The current situation and ways forward. *Epilepsia, 42*(1), 136–149.

Mgonela, V. A. (2010). *Obstacles and challenges faced by disabled women in employment opportunities in the public civil service in Tanzania: A case study of Dar es Salaam.* (Masters in Women's Law). Harare: University of Zimbabwe.

Morgan, H. (2012). The social model of disability as a threshold concept: Troublesome knowledge and liminal spaces in social work education. *Social Work Education, 31*(2), 215–226. doi:10.1080/02615479.2012.644964

Mtetwa, E. (2011). Policy dimensions of exclusion: Disability as charity and not right in Zimbabwe. *Indian Journal of Social Work, 72*(3), 381–398.

Mtetwa, E. (2016). Disability at the crossroads: The culture of exclusion and the 2013 constitution for Zimbabwe. *Journal of Social Development in Africa, 31*(2), 25–48.

Mugumbate J., Riphagenn H., & Gathara R. (2017). The role of social workers in the social management of epilepsy in Africa. In M. Gray (Ed.), *The handbook of social work and social development practice in Africa* (pp. 168–180). London: Routledge.

Murimi, P. (2013, November 2). Workplace a no-go area for people with disabilities. *Chronicle.* Retrieved June 12, 2017 from https://www.chronicle.co.zw/workplaces-a-no-go-area-for-people-with-disabilities/

Murungi, L. N., Mandlate, A., & Armah, B. (2013). Disability rights in the sub: Regional economic communities during 2011 and 2012. *African Disability Rights Yearbook, 1,* 375–383.

Mushi, D., Hunter, E., Mtuya, C., Mshana, G., Aris, E. & Walker, R. (2011). Social-cultural aspects of epilepsy in Kilimanjaro Region, Tanzania: Knowledge and experience among patients and carers. *Epilepsy and Behaviour, 20,* 338–343.

Mutanana, N., & Mutara, G. (2015). Health seeking behaviours of people with epilepsy in a rural community of Zimbabwe. *International Journal of Research in Humanities and Social Studies, 2*(2), 87–96.

Ndoye, N. F., Sow, A. D., Diop, A. G., Sessouma, B., Séne-Diouf, F., Boissy, L.,…, & Sander, J. W. A. S. (2005). Prevalence of epilepsy its treatment gap and knowledge, attitude and practice of its population in sub-urban Senegal an ILAE/IBE/WHO study. *Seizure: European Journal of Epilepsy, 14,* 106–111. doi:10.1016/j.seizure.2004.11.003

Newton, C. R., & Garcia, H. H. (2012). Epilepsy in poor regions of the world. *Lancet, 380*(9848), 1193–1201. doi:10.1016/s0140-6736(12)61381-6

Oliver, M. (1990). *The politics of disablement.* London: MacMillan.

Oliver, M. (2009). *Understanding disability: From theory to practice* (2nd ed.). New York: Palgrave Macmillan.

Oliver, M. (2013). *The social model of disablility: Thirty years on* (Vol. 28). Oxfordshire: Carfax International.

Peta, C., McKenzie, J., & Kathard, H. (2015). Voices from the periphery: A narrative study of the experiences of sexuality of disabled women in Zimbabwe. *Agenda, 29*(2), 66–76. doi:10.1080/10130950.2015.1050783

Quereshi, C., Standing, H. C., Swai, A., Hunter, E., Walker, R., & Owens, S. (2017). Barriers to access to education for young people with epilepsy in Northern Tanzania: A qualitative interview and focus group study involving teachers, parents and young people with epilepsy. *Epilepsy & Behavior, 72*, 145–149. doi:10.1016/j.yebeh.2017.04.005

Scott, D. F. (1992). The discovery of anti-epileptic drugs. *Journal of the History of the Neurosciences, 1*(2), 111–118. doi:10.1080/09647049209525522

Shorvon, S. (2009). *Epilepsy*. Oxford: Oxford University Press.

Shorvon, S. (2024). Should we use the word 'epilepsy'? *Epilepsy & Behavior, 157*, 109865. doi:10.1016/j.yebeh.2024.109865

Swain, J., & French, S. (2000). Towards an affirmation model of disability. *Disability & Society, 15*(4), 569–582. doi:10.1080/09687590050058189

Tuft, M., Nakken, K. O., & Kverndokk, K. (2017). Traditional folk beliefs on epilepsy in Norway and Sweden. *Epilepsy & Behavior, 71*, 104–107. doi:10.1016/j.yebeh.2017.03.032

United Nations (UN). (2006a). *Convention on the rights of persons with disabilities*. New York: UN.

United Nations (UN). (2006b). *Social justice in an open world: The role of the United Nations*. New York: UN.

Visagie, S., Scheffler, E., & Schneider, M. (2013). Policy implementation in wheelchair service delivery in a rural South African setting. *African Journal of Disability, 2*(1), 1–9.

Winkler, A. S., Mayer, M., Ombay, M., Mathias, B., Schmutzhard, E., & Jilek-Aall, L. (2009). Attitudes towards African traditional medicine and Christian spiritual healing regarding treatment of epilepsy in a rural community of northern Tanzania. *African Journal Traditional Complementary Alternative Medicine, 7*(2), 162–170.

World Health Organisation (WHO). (2015). *Sixty-Eighth World Health Assembly adopts resolution on epilepsy*. Retrieved December 13, 2016 from https://www.who.int/mental_health/neurology/epilepsy/resolution_68_20/en/

World Health Organisation (WHO). (2016). *Epilepsy*. Retrieved October 16, 2016 from https://www.who.int/mediacentre/factsheets/fs999/en/

World Health Organisation (WHO). (2022). Intersectoral global action plan on epilepsy and other neurological disorders 2022–2031 Retrieved November 3, 2022 from https://www.who.int/news/item/28-04-2022-draft-intersectoral-global-action-plan-on-epilepsy-and-other-neurological-disorders-2022-2031

World Health Organisation (WHO). (2024). Epilepsy. Retrieved from https://www.who.int/news-room/fact-sheets/detail/epilepsy

2 Competing interventions on treatment

In the Global South, interventions to epilepsy make it difficult to determine what is mainstay treatment and what is alternative, complementary or non-conventional healing practices. The main competing interventions are the cultural-religious and biopsychosocial. The World Health Organisation (WHO) (2000) defines cultural-religious interventions, which it terms 'traditional' as

> the sum total of the knowledge, skills and practices based on the theories, beliefs and experiences indigenous to different cultures, whether explicable or not, used in the maintenance of health, as well as in the prevention, diagnosis, improvement or treatment of physical and mental illnesses.
>
> (p. 1)

On the other hand, biopsychosocial interventions, consider physical health, mental well-being and social situation all together, using methods like medical clinical and technological diagnosis, pharmaceuticals, surgery, counselling and community support. Despite advances in diagnostic technology and antiepileptic medication, the medical treatment gap for epilepsy persists in the Global South due to competing treatments of epilepsy, and lack of access to affordable and readily available medical interventions. Up to 80–90% of people with epilepsy in the Global South are not on medical treatment (Adjaratou et al., 2015). This chapter uses results from a study done in Zimbabwe to exemplify competing interventions and illustrate the gaps that they create and the risks they pose to people with epilepsy.

African cultural-religious understandings

The population of people with epilepsy in Zimbabwe is estimated between 1% and 2% (Epilepsy Support Foundation [ESF], 2012). Mielke and Madzokere (2005) found a prevalence of 1.3% in a survey of the Hwedza District, which they conducted as part of the WHO-supported Global Campaign Against Epilepsy (GCAE). A national survey reported a disability prevalence of 7%, of which 2% of those surveyed had epilepsy. A study at Karanda Mission Hospital showed that epilepsy constituted 2.8% of hospital attendance during the period of the study (Vyas, Wong, Yang, Thistle, & Lee, 2016).

DOI: 10.4324/9781003602866-2

Indigenous understanding of epilepsy, emanating from African religion and culture sustain knowledge about epilepsy in Zimbabwe (Devlieger, Piachaud, Leung, & George, 1994; Mutanana & Mutara, 2015; Shoko, 2013). Despite colonisation by Christian and Islamic missionaries in the 15th century, Indigenous beliefs remain a key pillar of traditional Zimbabwean society. In African religion, God and ancestors work through healers—*n'anga* or *sangoma*—lending support to their faith-healing interventions (Andersson, 2002; Madzokere, 1997; Mutanana & Mutara, 2015; Vinga, 2014).

Research shows that in Zimbabwe epilepsy is interpreted as a supernatural condition inflicted by *vadzimu* (ancestors), *ngozi* (evil spirit) or witchcraft. Other explanations of epilepsy among the Shona are that seizures follow the phases of the moon, are genetic or resulted from objects in the stomach (ESF, 1992). Officials of the Shona religion, the *n'anga* (prophets, healers or seers) and *mhondoro* (spirit mediums) healed through inhalations, exorcism, rituals, incisions or body washing, then and now (Shoko, 2013).

In Zimbabwe, epilepsy is known as *pfari* (Shona) and *izifafa* (Ndebele) (Vinga, 2014) and is linked to *zvikwambo* (singular *chikwambo*), meaning goblin (also referred to as *zvidhoma, tokoroshi* and *zvishiri*), an evil or mischievous spirit; a playful or malicious elf; a frightful phantom; or a gnome. A *chikwambo* is an object imbued with magical powers that *n'anga* (healers) sell to people who believe that they will get rich quickly. Dube, Shoko and Haves (2011) explained that *zvikwambo* were often made of human body parts so the purchaser was usually urged to keep it secret from family members or within the family. Their continued efficacy depends on sacrifices, which became increasingly onerous. People regard the act of acquiring a *chikwambo* as witchcraft and believe that the ancestors or God would punish those who acquired riches in this evil way. *Zvikwambo* might be objects of misfortune or inexplicable riches, the latter attached to success stories or myths in Zimbabwean cultural tradition. To some, a *chikwambo* is the spirit of a dead person brought to life to slave for its owner. To others, it is an inanimate object that can transform into any creature. Other terms used are goblins, *zvidhoma, tokoroshi* and *zvishiri.*

Healers use various methods of spiritual healing in Zimbabwe. A popular method involves finding the witch responsible for supernatural interference and destroying his or her medicines or goblins by performing a spiritual ritual to render his or her powerless (Chavunduka, 1986). Ceremonial offerings as diverse as alcohol and animals are made to appease an angry God or ancestors, while the person with epilepsy, or family elders, pray for healing, deliverance and forgiveness (Mutanana & Mutara, 2015). Herbs might be swallowed, inhaled or inserted into the bloodstream through small cuts on the skin (ESF, 2012). Prescriptions include drinking, or bathing in, animal fat, blood, or urine or rubbing it on the skin or the wearing of red cloths and beads, or refraining from certain foods (Chavunduka, 1986). Healers often operate shrines, where people with epilepsy stay for treatment.

In Zimbabwe, Indigenous beliefs were institutionalised through the Traditional Medicines Practitioners Act, Witchcraft Suppression Act, and the Zimbabwe National African Traditional Healers' Association (ZINATHA), which was formed in 1980. However, despite efforts to improve traditional healing practices, they remain under researched, under regulated and ineffective. Most importantly, Indigenous beliefs have led to the denial of medical treatment for people with epilepsy, who spend time and resources for ineffective remedies.

Abrahamic (Judaism, Christianity and Islam) religious understandings

In Zimbabwe, Christian beliefs vary across Catholic, Protestant, Pentecostal and African churches though most religious adherents saw epilepsy as a punishment from God, a testing of one's faith by God, or a curse from an avenging evil spirit or witch (Chavunduka, 1986; Mutanana & Mutara, 2015). The treatment of epilepsy varies, though most churches advise adherents to have faith in God, read the bible, fast, pray and seek healing from prophets who use anointing oils, water, stones, and touch to heal the patient. Some churches entreated patients to wear bracelets with bible verses on them or a piece of cloth around the waist. In the past, prophets received tokens of appreciation if the healed could afford it, though nowadays they charged fees. Some religious healers run profitable shrines and retreats. Present-day prophecy in Zimbabwe is promoted through social and public media, where spiritual healers advertise their services and successes, and people are easily attracted to charismatic prophets, who permit diverse forms of payment, including church partnership or consultation fees; many advertised and sold lucrative anointing oils, holy water, towels, bangles, bracelets or other items thought to have healing powers (Chitando, Gunda, & Kügler, 2013). In the Pentecostal and African churches, this has become a huge business with some patients travelling to other African countries for spiritual healing (Chitando et al., 2013). Acceptance of medical treatment varies among Christian churches. The oldest African churches do not subscribe to medical treatment for spiritual conditions, though newer churches condoned the medical treatment of epilepsy (Shoko, 2013). Studies in other African countries observed similar beliefs and practices (Atadzhanov, Chomba, Haworth, Mbewe, & Birbeck, 2006; Mushi et al., 2011; Quereshi et al., 2017; Winkler et al., 2009).

In Islam, illness is a test of one's faith in Allah or an atonement for past sins (Al-Adawi et al., 2003; Almutairi, Ansari, Sami, & Baz, 2016; Daber-Taleh, Uwe, & Rösche, 2017; Mughees, 2006). Sickness is a wake-up call for enhanced spiritual connection with God through prayer, charity, meditation, forgiveness or remembrance of Allah and reading the Quran (Lawrence & Rozmus, 2001). Though God is their ultimate spiritual healer, Muslims, condone medical intervention (Ferguson, 2012). Zimbabwe's Muslim population is small, hence more information about Islam will be provided with reference to countries from the Middle East.

What is common to Indigenous African, and Islamic and Christian beliefs is the shared view that epilepsy is a supernatural condition wrought by God or the underworld, that is treatable only through faith, prayer, herbs or other medicines with the help of an *n'anga, jinn* or prophet.*** While the WHO appreciates that traditional treatments are used in the poorest countries, the organisation has expressed concerns about their safety, efficacy and quality, and the lack of research evidence to support their use (WHO, 2000). The WHO has consequently developed guidelines to support research of traditional treatments. However, a major problem with traditional treatments is their undervaluing of people with epilepsy. Belief systems work against the best interests of people with epilepsy, stigmatising them, and relegating them to the lowest ranks of society, in the process creating and sustaining social injustice against them, as the study on which this article is based, showed.

Both African cultural-religious understandings and Abrahamic (Judaism, Christianity and Islam) religious understandings of epilepsy have not provided a cure for epilepsy, nor have they improved the quality of life of people with epilepsy. As a result, society has continually looked for solutions to epilepsy. At the moment, biological, psychological and social interventions, backed by research, have provided the best remedy for most people with epilepsy (Mugumbate & Gray, 2017a, 2017b). However, this has increased competition of interventions.

Biopsychosocial interventions

Zimbabwe adopted a biopsychosocial approach to epilepsy a long time ago, and allowed this intervention to work alongside African cultural-religious and Abrahamic interventions. Using the biopsychosocial model, epilepsy is viewed as a neurological, psychological, mental health and disabling non-communicable condition. A medical approach uses diagnostics, pharmaceuticals or surgery to treat epilepsy. It emphasises the role of the individual in seeking and maintaining medical treatment. It is often supported by the psychological interventions that focus on the mind and behaviour. However, both medical and psychological interventions do not take into account of social and cultural factors that prevent people with epilepsy, in this instance, from accessing appropriate health services (Adjaratou et al., 2015). Social interventions take into account of the social, economic, cultural and political environment influencing people's health choices (Mugumbate, Riphagenn, & Gathara, 2017). It focuses on the way in which these broader factors lead to health inequalities and marginalises groups of people with less power in society, such as people with disabilities, older people, and women and children, from accessing the services they need. The WHO (2000) has for long promoted a biopsychosocial approach because it addresses the broader factors hampering access to medical treatment for people with epilepsy (Oliver, 2013). The WHO introduced the biopsychosocial model (often referred to as the Model of Functioning and Disability) and the International Classification of Functioning, Disability and Health (ICF) (WHO, 2000). The WHO model views disability from three perspectives: *biological*–physical ability (impairments of bodily functions and structures), *psychological*–cognitive activity limitations and participation restrictions) and social-environmental factors. Given the medical, social and cultural challenges faced by people with epilepsy in Zimbabwe, the biopsychosocial model appears to cover all but one factor needed for epilepsy management; it omits highly important spiritual factors. This is possibly why the uptake of medical treatment has been persistently low in Africa in general and Zimbabwe in particular since the ongoing reliance on ineffective traditional healing practices is overlooked.

How the competition happens

If epilepsy is noticed in the family or community, the usual point of call is the cultural, religious or spiritual healer (Mugumbate & Gray, 2017a, 2017b; Mugumbate et al., 2022). The healer will do diagnosis and offer options for 'cure' and the patients go back home. Naturally, seizure will stop because all seizures are temporary. This gives the family relief until the seizures come again. They may go back to the healer for more advanced treatment or seek another healer. Several months may pass before going to the clinic to see a nurse or doctor. The treatment guidelines in Zimbabwe allow nurses to do a clinical diagnosis for epilepsy and initiate treatment, depending on the type of seizures. Otherwise, they diagnose and refer to the next level of health service where more experienced nurses or a doctor is found. Meanwhile, the patient may still be getting healing from healers. The healers often dissuade people with epilepsy from seeking clinical treatment, while nurses and doctors often tell patients not to visit healers. Initial medical treatment may work and the patient may stop taking medicines thinking that epilepsy has been cured, and also respecting advice from healers. Or if they continue taking medicines and there are side effects, which is common, there will be a reason to stop the medication, a trend common in resource-limited settings (Mugumbate et al., 2022). Defaulting medication may result from side effects, lack of money to buy them or go to a clinic or hospital to collect free medicines. If medical treatment fails to control seizures or there are side effects, the patient is referred to the next level, where they will see a specialist. There are very few specialists in Zimbabwe, for both children and adults, as in many countries of the Global South (Mugumbate & Zimba, 2018). The specialist may request to change medicine to an expensive one which government does not offer for free, and may also ask for further technology-aided diagnostics. Often, the patient does not afford both, and therefore, the goal of tertiary management is not achieved (Mugumbate & Gray, 2021).

Doctors and nurses, at any stage of the process, may refer patients to other health workers, for example, psychologists and psychiatrists and allied health workers, for example, counsellors and social workers. In other circumstances, they refer to healers, though this is not considered standard practice. Very few hospitals have social workers, so the referral is often to a non-government organisation, such as the Epilepsy Support Foundation (ESF), the Epilepsy Resource Centre Zimbabwe or other health and disability groups and networks. Besides patients who visit through referrals, the ESF and ERCZ also get visitors who respond to their awareness programmes, mainly during national epilepsy week, Epilepsy Stripes Week and International Epilepsy Day (Mugumbate et al., 2023).

To gain a deeper understanding of how the competition for treatment unfolds, a study was done in Zimbabwe. The qualitative study involved 30 in-depth interviews with people with epilepsy in Harare, Zimbabwe's capital. The purposively selected sample comprised 13 males and 17 females aged between 15 and 64 years. Data were analysed using N-Vivo, a computer-assisted qualitative data-analysis package. A focus group discussion was held with seven service providers at the ESF, a private (voluntary) organisation found in 1990 to provide psychological, educational, economic, social, spiritual and medical support to people with epilepsy.

Treatments used by participants

Most participants (n = 26) used several methods of treatment before accessing medical treatment, while others mixed traditional and medical treatments. Traditional treatments comprised AIR and Christian methods offered by family members, prophets, congregants, herbalists, traditional healers or spiritualists. AIR methods included ancestral prayer, and spiritual and herbal healing, while Christian methods included faith healing, prayer, fasting and use of mantles. Service providers reported that some people with epilepsy with whom they had worked used Eastern traditional medicines from China and Korea. None of the participants used Islamic methods. Yet others alternated traditional and medical treatments, with a view to finding an effective means for seizure control. As regards the reasons for using traditional treatments, Derry (not real name) said 'we thought it was to do with family spirits' and Lameck remarked that 'I had a seizure [when I was about to get a good job], someone bewitched me. Derry's employer, and friends in Botswana and South Africa, where he worked, just believed it was caused by evil spirits and needed prophets'. Similarly, Lameck sought traditional treatment because he believed he was bewitched. Derry, Lameck and many other participants sought traditional treatments because they believed epilepsy was a supernatural condition. When asked about the benefits of traditional remedies, participants said they were cheaper, readily available, better understood, and, as Mucha explained, 'that is the way it is done'. Other participants, such as Saru, said that people did not know that epilepsy was a treatable medical condition. In reference to her early treatment experiences, Saru said, 'I did not know about [medical] treatment. I used to try everything'. This included several years of unsuccessful faith healing, herbal treatments and traditional cleansing.

Indigenous methods of treatment

> They then took me to several n'angas, some as far as neighbouring Mozambique [neighbouring country which is 200 kilometres away]. When this failed [to stop seizures], they took me back home and prepared a ceremonial brew, where a cow was killed and the meat was eaten without salt. Most senior members of the extended family were present. Again, nothing worked.
>
> (Agnell)

Agnella recounted how paraphernalia for witches was destroyed by a healer at their home, including a calabash filled with blood and decorated with colourful beards. Munya and Ashley described experiences almost similar to Agnel's. Gab and Kocho underwent ritual cleansing at their homes and visited spiritualists for cleansing. They said this was the usual cultural practice in their communities.

Christian treatments

> My husband, a … church reverend, prayed for me for days. He gave me white clothes to wear and holy water to drink. When this did not stop seizures, we

went to other members of the church. These were more senior prophets, but nothing helped. They recommended more fasting and prayer and an all-night prayer at our home. My husband brought a prophet from another church who said the problem of seizures was a result of a spirit coming from my paternal family. The seizures continued and I think I was mad at that time.

(Agnel)

Other participants described experiences that included night church vigils, prayer, fasting, and use of holy water, oil, mantles, and wearing pieces of cloth. Participants visited *n'angas* in faraway places to get treatment. Saru said: 'We tried all means for me to get treatment. At one point we left our car in the bush when we had visited herbalists in Nyanga. Somewhere very far'. The area she and her family had gone to for treatment was several kilometres away.

Herbal medicines and mhiko *treatment*

What assisted me was herbal tea provided at church. It's a spiritual drink from church. … It's given by prophets. At times it's salt water. I used it until a friend told me about this [ESF] organisation.

(Gab)

Herbal medicines and *mhiko* (a covenant between the healer and the person with epilepsy) were used for both church-based and Indigenous methods of treatment. Other participants used roots, leaves, tree bark juice or concoctions made from animal products. Lameck had burnt incense, that is, he put herbs in a burning fire and breathed in the fumes or put herbs in hot water and inhaled the vapour under a blanket. Lameck and Mambe had a *mhiko* of not to eat chicken and beans. Lameck was given a piece of cloth (as a *mhiko*) to wear around his waist, to wade off evil. The piece of cloth was not to be removed under any circumstances.

Transition to medical treatment

Until about March, I saw this old man in Mhondoro who gave us some concoctions. It stopped for about a month and the seizures started.

(Lameck)

However, after trying prophets, *n'anga*, and other traditional methods, Lameck's seizures did not stop. He visited local hospitals but his epilepsy was never diagnosed. Each time he went, he received bandages and painkillers. Later, he was advised by his aunt about medical treatment available at the ESF, whereafter he had sought medical treatment. Most participants had eventually sought medical treatment at the ESF following the failure of prolonged traditional treatments. Derry and Mucha said their seizures had been briefly controlled with traditional treatments, but the medical treatment had led to permanent seizure control.

Views of service providers

Service providers agreed that contrary to professional health ethics, some medical personnel persuaded people with epilepsy to seek traditional treatment, arguing that epilepsy was a spiritual and cultural condition. They said this was one of the reasons participants sought traditional treatments. They (service providers) added that some people with epilepsy used Eastern medicine from China and Korea, including herbal medicines, and chiropractic and acupressure natural therapies. Asked why reliance on traditional treatments was high, service providers said communities lacked correct knowledge of epilepsy and medical treatment services were beyond the reach of most people with epilepsy; hence, they opted for cheaper and readily available traditional treatments. Focus Group Participant 5 said participants expected to be seizure free quickly, something even medical treatment does not achieve in most instances. This resulted in them using several treatment options.

The service providers highlighted that epilepsy management fell under the Mental Health Unit of the Ministry of Health and the Disability Unit of the Social Welfare Department. However, both units were understaffed, under resourced and underfinanced nor did they have a specific policy to deal with epilepsy. The resources for nationwide awareness initiatives were lacking, and the government had not prioritised epilepsy in the allocation of public resources. Yet, service providers agreed that each time they promoted epilepsy awareness, the number of people coming 'out of the shadows' to visit ESF for medical treatment increased. Without government support, service providers pointed out that people with epilepsy ended up going to organisations like the ESF, for help yet the organisations had limited capacity to deal with the volume of people seeking support.

A deeper understanding of competing treatments

Medical treatment is the alternative not main intervention

Based on the views of participants reported in this chapter, medical treatment was complementary or alternative to cultural, spiritual and religious remedies for epilepsy in the first years of seizure onset. However, participants' experiences showed that their seizures were not controlled with traditional treatments, despite several years of using them. This is a common occurrence in Africa (Mielke & Madzokere, 2005) but the practice leads to delayed medical treatment and ongoing debilitating seizures. The overreliance on traditional treatments is as much a factor of erroneous beliefs as of their ready availability within the community. Traditional healing is a well-embedded social, religious, spiritual and cultural institution and an opaque industry that generates livelihoods for its practitioners. Traditional treatments prices vary, but in most cases, each client has a package that suits them. The prices are negotiable and terms for payment are available. Payment does not necessarily need to be cash; it could be anything from livestock, grain, furniture or services.

Poor medical services reduced the treatment gap

Use of traditional treatments was compounded by the lack of availability of less costly medical treatment. Zimbabwe has a strong infrastructure of public health services in urban areas but service quality is erratic; hospitals are overcrowded and under-resourced. Reliable private services were available but were expensive. In Zimbabwe, there is no strong community health workforce educating communities about the ease with which epilepsy can be treated if properly understood as a neurological condition. Delayed treatment, or lack of access to medical intervention, led not only to social problems relating to education and unemployment, but also to psychological and mental health problems and social isolation. People with epilepsy in the reported study had received treatment and social support from the ESF in Harare but the majority of people living with epilepsy in Zimbabwe are severely disadvantaged by the prevalence of ignorance and absence of appropriate resources, especially in rural areas (Mielke & Madzokere, 2005). The dire economic situation in Zimbabwe does little to improve the situation. The solutions to increasing uptake of medical treatment lie in affordable healthcare, and community education and awareness (Mielke & Madzokere, 2005), roles the government of Zimbabwe was not adequately playing. As this study showed, awareness of epilepsy as a treatable condition increased treatment uptake. However, focus group participants said the resources for nationwide awareness initiatives were nonexistent, and government had not prioritised epilepsy in the allocation of public resources.

Shortcomings of both interventions

This reported study showed that traditional treatment services in Zimbabwe had serious flaws: traditional medicines were unregulated, there was no guarantee of success and the institutions to monitor the whole system were lax. The Traditional Medical Practitioners Act regulated though its Council had weak implementation and monitoring mechanism. A stronger regulatory framework was needed to avoid unnecessary delays in medical treatment. On a positive note, traditional treatment is community based and it has potential to be used to mobilise communities for epilepsy awareness. The results of the study exposed the challenges of accessing medical treatment for people with epilepsy in Zimbabwe. Participants reported that they received poor treatment, including delayed diagnosis when they finally visited clinics for medical treatment. Some reported that they had medical treatment plans that were not reviewed for lengthy periods of time, despite failed seizure control. This opened room for them to go back to traditional treatments.

Medical treatment has potential to improve quality of life and reduce the burden of epilepsy

It is well known that a lack of access to antiepileptic medication leads to disability, economic loss and a poor quality of life for people with epilepsy (Hajjioui & Fourtassi, 2014; Mugumbate, 2017). Quality of life in epilepsy refers to how well someone with epilepsy feels and functions in daily life. It includes aspects like physical health, mental well-being, social relationships and the ability to do everyday activities. Factors such as how often seizures happen, side effects from medication, and support from friends and family can all play a role. Improving quality of life often means finding effective treatments, managing stress and making healthy lifestyle choices, all of which can help individuals live more fulfilling lives (WHO, 2022).

Seizure frequency or severity is a crucial factor in determining the quality of life for individuals with epilepsy in Zimbabwe and similar resource-limited settings. Frequent or severe seizures can lead to physical injuries, increased anxiety and a general sense of instability (Mugumbate, 2010). This unpredictability can affect daily routines and limit participation in social activities, making individuals feel isolated. Additionally, a lack of access to antiepileptic medication exacerbates this issue, as untreated seizures significantly diminish confidence and the ability to engage with the world (Hajjioui & Fourtassi, 2014).

The side effects of epilepsy medications can also impact quality of life, especially in resource-limited settings where access to a range of treatment options may be limited. Many people experience fatigue, dizziness, weight gain or mood changes, which can hinder daily functioning and overall well-being. These side effects may discourage adherence to treatment, leading to more seizures and further complications. Finding the right medication with manageable side effects is essential for improving daily life and allowing individuals to feel more like themselves (Hajjioui & Fourtassi, 2014).

The functional impact of epilepsy can significantly influence an individual's work life in Zimbabwe. Some people may find it challenging to maintain steady employment due to the unpredictability of seizures or the effects of medications (Mugumbate, 2017). Others might experience improved work performance when seizures are well controlled, allowing them to contribute effectively and pursue career goals. Support from employers and understanding colleagues can further enhance job satisfaction and overall quality of life.

The well-being of caregivers is another important aspect of quality of life in epilepsy, particularly in resource-limited settings where support systems may be less robust. When individuals with epilepsy receive effective treatment, it not only benefits them but also improves the lives of their caregivers. Reduced seizure frequency and severity can lessen the emotional and physical strain on family members, leading to better relationships and a more supportive home environment (Hajjioui & Fourtassi, 2014). This improvement allows caregivers to focus on their own needs and well-being, as well as the needs of the individual with epilepsy.

People with epilepsy can still contribute meaningfully to their households and communities. When seizures are well managed, individuals can take on responsibilities at home, participate in community events and engage in volunteer work. This sense of contribution enhances self-esteem and helps foster a sense of belonging, which is vital for overall happiness and life satisfaction (WHO, 2022).

Relationships can be deeply affected by epilepsy, both positively and negatively. Seizures and their unpredictability can strain friendships and romantic partnerships, often leading to feelings of isolation. However, with effective management of the condition, individuals can build and maintain strong, supportive relationships. Open communication about epilepsy can help friends and loved ones understand the condition better, fostering empathy and support (Hajjioui & Fourtassi, 2014).

Having future plans and ambitions is essential for anyone's sense of purpose, and this is especially true for individuals with epilepsy in Zimbabwe. The fear of seizures can sometimes hinder aspirations, whether in education, career or personal goals. However, with effective treatment and support, many people with epilepsy can pursue their dreams and make long-term plans, fostering hope and motivation in their lives (Mugumbate & Gray, 2017a, 2017b).

Overall health is a key component of quality of life for those with epilepsy, particularly in resource-limited settings like Zimbabwe. Managing the condition often involves maintaining a healthy lifestyle, including regular exercise, a balanced diet and sufficient sleep. These factors can positively influence both physical and mental health, reducing the risk of additional health issues and improving overall well-being. Staying active and healthy contributes to greater resilience in facing the challenges of living with epilepsy (Mugumbate, 2010).

Conclusion

As shown by the examples from Zimbabwe, the choice of treatments for epilepsy is influenced by beliefs and the availability of accessible medical treatment. Further, there are multiple barriers to initiating and sustaining medical treatment for people with epilepsy, resulting in sustained use of religious, cultural and spiritual treatments, even when they are ineffective. The problem of a huge medical treatment gap does not seem to lie in individual choices but in the failure of people with epilepsy to have the resources needed for medical treatment. The government needs to make resources available for more epilepsy awareness programmes to promote modern understandings and treatments; service providers need training to enhance the professionalism of the support services they provide; and medical treatment needs to be made affordable and readily available. In the end, research on best ways to integrate traditional treatments with modern medical treatments is desirable as results of such research could be used to increase seizure control, the goal of both treatments. Given the important findings relating to persistent cultural, spiritual and religious understandings, further research would need to focus on a biopsychosocial spiritual model of epilepsy to fully encompass the influence of spiritual beliefs and practices that are a key feature of all parts of resource-limited settings.

References

Adjaratou, D., Toure, K., Ndeye, F., Basee-Faye, A., Marieme, S., Ndiaga, M., et al. (2015). Prevalence and risk factors of nonadherence to epilepsy treatment in Dakar, Senegal. *African and Middle East Epilepsy Journal, 4(1)*, 16–20.

Al-Adawi, S., Al-Salmy, H., Martin, R. G., Al-Naamani, A., Prabhakar, S., Deleu, D., & Dorvlo, A. S. (2003). Patient's perspective on epilepsy: Self-knowledge among Omanis. *Seizure, 12(1)*, 11–18.

Almutairi, M. A., Ansari, T., Sami, W., & Baz, S. (2016). Public knowledge and attitudes toward epilepsy in Majmaah. *Journal of Neurosciences in Rural Practice, 7*(4), 499–503. doi:10.4103/0976-3147.188622

Andersson, J. A. (2002). Sorcery in the era of 'Henry IV': Kinship, mobility and mortality in Buhera District, Zimbabwe. *Journal of the Royal Anthropological Institute, 8*(3), 425–449.

Atadzhanov, M., Chomba, E., Haworth, A., Mbewe, E., & Birbeck, G. L. (2006). Knowledge, attitudes, behaviors, and practices regarding epilepsy among Zambian clerics. *Epilepsy & Behavior, 9*(1), 83–88. doi:http://dx.doi.org/10.1016/j.yebeh.2006.03.012

Chitando, E., Gunda, M. R., & Kügler, J. (2013). Introduction. In E. Chitando, M.R. Gunda & J. Kügler (Eds.), Prophets, profits and the Bible in Zimbabwe (pp. 1–14). Bamberg: University of Bamberg Press.

Chavunduka, G. L. (1986). Realties of witchcraft. Harare: University of Zimbabwe.

Daber-Taleh, S., Uwe, W., & Rösche, J. (2017). Knowledge and attitude towards epilepsy among students of economics in Herat, Afghanistan. *Neurology Asia, 22*(1), 1–8.

Devlieger, P., Piachaud, J., Leung, P., & George, N. (1994). Coping with epilepsy in Zimbabwe and the Midwest, USA. *International Journal of Rehabilitation Research, 17*(3), 251–264.

Dube, L., Shoko, T., & Haves, S. (2011). *African initiatives in healing ministry*. Pretoria: Unisia Press.

Epilepsy Support Foundation. (2012). About epilepsy 2012. Harare: Epilepsy Support Foundation.

Ferguson, C. (2012). Perceptions of epilepsy in Morocco, seen by an American Neuroscientist. *North African and Middle East Epilepsy Journal, 1*(4), 4–7.

Hajjioui, A., & Fourtassi, M. (2014). Epilepsy and disability. *North African and Middle East Epilepsy Journal, 3*(5), 17–19.

Lawrence, P., & Rozmus, C. (2001). Culturally sensitive care of the Muslim patient. *Journal of Transcultural Nursing, 12*(3), 228–233.

Madzokere, C. (1997). Life experiences of people with epilepsy. A study of highfield high density residential area in Harare, Zimbabwe. *EPICADEC News (biannual newsletter of Foundation Epilepsy Care Developing Countries, 10*(97), 19–21.

Mielke, J., & Madzokere, C. (2005). Epilepsy care in rural Zimbabwe: A global campaign against epilepsy project. *Epilepsia, 46*, 347.

Mughees, A. (2006). Better caring for Muslim patients. *World of Irish Nursing and Midwifery, 14(7)*, 24–15.

Mugumbate, J., & Gray, M. (2017a). Competing traditional and medical treatments of epilepsy in Harare, Zimbabwe. *African and Middle East Journal of Epilepsy, 6(2)*, 1–9.

Mugumbate, J., & Gray, M. (2017b). Individual resilience as a strategy to counter employment barriers for people with epilepsy in Zimbabwe. *Epilepsy and Behaviour.* March, 74C, 154-160. doi:10.1016/j.yebeh.2017.06.018

Mugumbate, J., & Gray, M. (2021). Employment rights for people with epilepsy in Zimbabwe: A social justice perspective. In V. Sewpaul, L. Kreitzer & T. Raniga (Eds.), *The tensions between culture and human rights. Emancipatory social work and Afrocentricity in a Global World* (pp 81–99). Calgary: University of Calgary Press.

Mugumbate, J., Riphagenn, H., & Gathara, R. (2017). The role of social workers in the social management of epilepsy in Africa. In M. Gray (Ed.), *The handbook of social work and social development in Africa* (pp. 168–180). London: Routledge.

Mugumbate, J., & Zimba, A. (2018). Epilepsy in Africa: Past, present, and future. *Epilepsy & Behavior, 7*, 239–241. doi:10.1016/j.yebeh.2017.10.009

Mugumbate, J. R. (2010). *Global Campaign Against Epilepsy (GCAE) Zimbabwe report.* Harare: Epilepsy Support Foundation.

Mugumbate, J. R., Kissani, N., Acevedo, K., Mugumbate, C., Janneh, A., Lilia Núñez-Orozco, L., Mauricio, O. A., & Ibrahim, E. A. A. (2022). First Aid (FA) and First Guidance (FG) for epilepsy seizures: Key considerations and recommendations for developing regions of the world. *Journal of Social Issues in Non-Communicable Conditions & Disability, 1*(1), 11–24.

Mugumbate, R. (2017). Disability, employment, and social justice. Employment experiences of people with epilepsy in Harare, Zimbabwe. Doctor of Philosophy thesis. University of Newcastle.

Mugumbate, R., Klevor, R., Aguirre, M. O., Massi, G.D., Yaqoob, N., Acevedo, K., Yewnetu, E., Kanyabutembo, C., Ibrahim, E. A. A., Boutadghart, S., Janneh, A., & Kissani, N. (2023). Epilepsy awareness days, weeks, and months: Their roles in the fight against epilepsy and the intersectoral global action plan on epilepsy and other neurological disorders, *Epilepsy & Behavior, 148*, 109457, doi:10.1016/j.yebeh.2023.109457

Mutanana, N., & Mutara, G. (2015). Health seeking behaviours of people with epilepsy in a rural community of Zimbabwe. *International Journal of Research in Humanities and Social Studies 2*(2), 87–96.

Oliver, M. (2013). *The social model of disablility: Thirty years on.* Oxfordshire: Carfax International Publishers.

Quereshi, C., Standing, H. C., Swai, A., Hunter, E., Walker, R., & Owens, S. (2017). Barriers to access to education for young people with epilepsy in Northern Tanzania: A qualitative interview and focus group study involving teachers, parents and young people with epilepsy. *Epilepsy & Behavior, 72*, 145–149. doi:10.1016/j.yebeh.2017.04.005

Shoko, T. (2013). Shona traditional religion and medical practices: Methodological approaches to religious phenomena. *Journal of Religion in Africa, 43*(3), 360–380.

Vinga, A. (2014, 27 July). Half a million people in Zimbabwe live with epilepsy. *The Sunday Mail.* Retrieved December 12, 2015 from http://sundaymail.co.zw/half-a-million-people-in-Zimbabwe-live-with-epilepsy/

Vyas, M. V., Wong, A., Yang, J. M., Thistle, P., & Lee, L. (2016). The spectrum of neurological presentations in an outpatient clinic of rural Zimbabwe. Journal of the Neurological Sciences, 362, 263–265. doi:10.1016/j.jns.2016.01.065

Wehbe-Alamah, H. (2008). Bridging generic and professional care practices for Muslim patients through use of Leininger's culture care models. *Contemporary Nursing, 28*(1), 83–97.

Winkler, A. S., Mayer, M., Ombay, M., Mathias, B., Schmutzhard, E., & Jilek-Aall, L. (2009). Attitudes towards African traditional medicine and Christian spiritual healing regarding treatment of epilepsy in a rural community of northern Tanzania. *African Journal Traditional Complementary Alternative Medicine, 7*(2), 162–170.

World Health Organisation (WHO). (2000). *General guidelines for methodologies on research and evaluation of traditional medicine.* Geneva: WHO.

3 Brain health, prevention and determinants of epilepsy

A major theme in the management of epilepsy is prevention of first-onset epilepsy, which is about avoiding people from developing epilepsy in the first place. According to WHO (2022, 2024), about 25% of epilepsies can be prevented. The challenge though is that not all causes of epilepsy are known, making it impossible to prevent them. Nonetheless, there are strategies that could be employed to reduce the risk of developing epilepsy. A difference should be understood between preventing epilepsy and preventing seizures. Since epilepsy is the condition that results in seizures, this chapter is about preventing epilepsy. Preventing seizures happens when a person already has epilepsy, hence this chapter is not about preventing seizures from recurring. Seizures are prevented from recurring by treatment, and other means and they can also be prevented from recurring by avoiding triggers. This chapter will begin by conceptualising prevention and brain health. This will include the benefits of prevention and maintaining brain health. It will then discuss individual strategies, followed by family, community, environmental, societal and global strategies. Examples of prevention will be provided at each level, as well as potential challenges.

Brain health

Brain health is about ensuring the cognitive and physical well-being of the brain to ensure optimal memory, attention and problem-solving abilities. If there is injury to the brain, its structural and functional integrity is impacted. In the previous chapter, the electrical theory of epilepsy was introduced. The thesis of the theory is that epilepsy results from electrical activity in the brain. But how does this happen?

Information box 3.1   How seizures happen—the electrical theory

When a person's brain is healthy, small amounts of electricity are supplied to the brain in a controlled and balanced manner resulting in normal thinking, movement, and feelings. When there is more, excessive or misfiring electricity, all this becomes abnormal, causing uncontrolled movement, thinking or feelings, or in short, seizures. Think about a light bulb connected to a

---

DOI: 10.4324/9781003602866-3

battery or electricity. If the flow of power is steady, the light does not flick but if there is too much or the power is cutting, the bulb may flicker but if the power steadies, it comes back to normal. If there is excessive power, the bulb may burn. This is what happens with seizures. Electricity in the brain is transmitted by neurons which may misfire, send excessive current or send it in an unusual pattern. This is one reason electricity gets disturbed in the brain. The other reasons are body chemical imbalances, brain injury or damage and genes. Brain injury or damage can result from infections or head trauma, factors that can also result in brain tumours. Developmental disorders, stroke and neurodegenerative diseases can result in epilepsy. Some causes are unknown.

Kakooza-Mwesige, Katabira and Kaggwa (2015b), Lüders and Klem (2018), Engel and Pitkänen (2016). Kwan and Brodie (2015). Scharfman and Sollas (2017) and Gloor and Moffat (2018).

Information box 3.2　How pigs can cause epilepsy

Pig meat or pork may carry a tapeworm called taenia solium. This worm lives in pig flesh and can be consumed by humans if the meat is not well cooked. If consumed, the worm travels to parts of the body, including the brain, where it deposits some larva or small bags containing fluids. The cysts block normal electrical activity in the rain, cause the rain to swell or alter chemical imbalance resulting in neurological symptoms, including seizures, headaches and altered thinking or in medical terms, neurocysticercosis. Neurocysticercosis is very common in East Africa, especially Uganda and South Sudan. The prevalence of epilepsy is also high in these areas as a result. Conditions that promote taenia solium in these countries include unhygienic food practices, pig-rearing practices, poor sanitation, limited access to health care, inadequate health education and poverty results if low economic means to rear pigs in healthy environments and improve human sanitation.

Kakooza-Mwesige, Kaggwa and Katabira (2015a), Kariuki, Njenga and Karanja (2017), Gikonyo, Mureithi and Mwaura (2018), and Ndagije, Mufunda and Kizza (2019).

Everyday situations that impact brain health

There are many everyday situations that could potentially result in epilepsy. If in his or her gene, a parent has a gene susceptible to epilepsy, this gene may be passed on to the foetus and they are born with genes that may result in epilepsy. For unborn babies, exposing them to head trauma can result in epilepsy, for example, if the mother's tummy is hard in a human violence incident. Trauma to the foetus can also result from the mother falling hard on their tummy or a cow hitting her tummy. If the mother smokes or drinks alcohol, this may impact the feotus's chemical imbalance. If the baby inherits genes that are not susceptible to epilepsy, and again survives trauma while in the womb, there will still be another hurdle. During birth, the process may be prolonged or difficult due to the size of the cavity, the mother or the baby. A prolonged labour may result in developmental delay and seizures while a difficult labour may result in head trauma. Newborn babies are susceptible to infections, for example, meningitis, encephalitis, brain abscess, neurocysticercosis, Human Immunodeficiency Virus/Acquired Immunodeficiency Syndrome (HIV/AIDS) and herpes simplex virus infection. Further, lead, mercury and organophosphates may cause epilepsy. When the child starts moving around, injuries may result from moving objects such as machines and animals such as horses or donkeys. When they become active young children, the risk of head trauma from tree climbing, bicycle riding, sports and work activities is high. If they survive this, in teenagerhood, they can be exposed to drugs and alcohol, which may have disastrous effects to the brain, including epilepsy if consumed to excess. In adulthood, the risk of human violence through hand lighting, weapons and beating is high, and women often suffer more from this. There is also risk of head trauma at work, in farms, mines, transport, construction and other industries. Riding *boda boda* (motorcycles as they are called in East Africa), scooters or mopeds (motorcycles as they are called in Asia) without helmets exposes riders to head injury. A lot of road accidents result from drunk driving and over speeding, which are easily avoidable.

Strategies to prevent epilepsy

As noted above, preventing epilepsy is possible; however, for epilepsies whose cause is not known, it is not possible to prevent them. A key strategy is to maintain brain health. This can be achieved by living and maintaining a safe lifestyle that prevents head injuries. When riding, wearing helmets is a simple strategy. Other strategies include reducing speed and maintaining reasonable loads. Road and traffic rules that protect riders are required, as often, riders are hit by other traffic. An example of such a rule is to regulate the distance traffic can keep from riders to avoid dangerous situations such as overtaking. The age of rides should also be regulated by licencing at the most appropriate age.

Most infections can be controlled easily by maintaining clean environments and eating clean foods. A case in point is the taenia solium tapeworm which causes neurocysticercosis. The tapeworm can be prevented by rearing pigs in healthy environments and by thoroughly cooking pork before consumption. In Africa, and other parts of the world HIV has been successfully prevented by not having sex with an infected partner and using condoms if a partner is infected or you are unsure of their HIV status. More importantly, abstinence from sex is a sure way to prevent infection. At the societal level, reducing early onset of sex has proved helpful in Eswatini. Sharing needles used to inject the body with medicines and drugs increase risk of HIV, and this should be avoided. These strategies apply to preventing herpes simplex virus too. Meningitis is caused by meningococcal, pneumococcal and hib bacteria which can all be vaccinated against. Encephalitis is caused by mosquitoes such as the West Nile virus and other animals, so, avoid mosquito bites and contact with animals that cause it is preventative measure. Encephalitis can also result from measles, mumps, and rubella, conditions that can be vaccinated against. A brain abscess or pockets of pus result from bacteria, fungi or pathogens that invade the brain from other infected parts of the body, mainly teeth. This is preventable by preventing body wounds and infections in the first place or treating them early. Finally, getting early intervention and treatment for these infections is helpful to prevent seizures.

Pregnancy preparation and prenatal care are important strategies to prevent epilepsy for the foetus and newborn babies. Pregnancy preparation involves all practices that prepare the to-be-pregnant mother to be safe to the foetus when conception happens while prenatal care is about the practices that remove or reduce harm to the foetus. The health of the mother is important, and it should be monitored before and after conception. When conception happens, the size of the foetus needs to be monitored. Risk of traumatic incidences, for example domestic violence, should be monitored. Drugs, alcohol, tobacco and other harmful substances during pregnancy increase the risk of epilepsy for the baby. In resource-limited settings, unwanted pregnancies force some people into attempting unsafe abortions using chemicals or physical methods. This is very dangerous to the foetus. This can be avoided by having planned pregnancies inside marriages. Delivery should always be monitored by experienced of trained people and should happen in a safe environment, where emergency help is assured if needed. In resource-limited settings, labour services are provided in villages by experienced women; however, they are often not able to deal with emergencies. Labour services are also provided in primary care facilities where trained maternity workers or midwives are found; however, in some remote settings, these primary care facilities are not well connected to the secondary and tertiary health systems to cater for emergencies.

As alluded to earlier, genetics is one of the causes of epilepsy. Having genetic counselling can be useful in preventing the condition. If there is epilepsy in the family tree, a genetic counsellor will interpret what that may mean to the health of other offsprings of the family, and the options available to them. They will provide information about what could be potentially inherited, and how it can be managed. In other cases, doctors can recommend genetic testing, which the counsellor may help interpret in ways that are easy to understand.

When neurological symptoms first appear, it is important to have early diagnosis and treatment to reduce the impact. In the example of neurocysticercosis provided earlier, continued exposure to epilepsy-causing worms can result in more damage to the brain, resulting in more and frequent seizures which are difficult to treat. Further, more family members can get infected because they are in the same environment, and they are consuming the same pork which is contaminated. Another advantage with early diagnosis is that a more accurate understanding of the condition is obtained to help make treatment more effective.

Chronic conditions such as blood pressure, diabetes, stroke, obesity and neurodegenerative diseases such as dementia, make people prone to epilepsy, therefore managing these conditions with proper treatment prevents epilepsy. For people with these chronic conditions, regular monitoring, medication adherence and lifestyle modifications are recommended.

Accidents during work or traffic accidents are usually always avoidable by observing work health and safety procedures. Drivers need to never drive after consuming more than a glass of alcohol or after taking intoxicating substances. Traffic speeds need to be low to suit the conditions. Seat belts and helmets have been shown to save lives, and this should be a must. Governments should ensure that roads are safe throughout the year and that traffic rules are observed and monitored.

Older adults are prone to multiple chronic conditions, the most common being neurodegenerative diseases which include Alzheimer's, Parkinson's and dementia. Managing these conditions in adults will help reduce the risk of them developing epilepsy. However, in resource-limited settings, old age may be viewed from a spiritual lens, resulted in delayed treatment of chronic conditions or no treatment of all.

Strategies at the global level can be very useful in setting standards and preventing outbreaks of infections. This work is usually led by the WHO through its regional offices. Global efforts were instrumental in reducing HIV, as an example. If more of this kind of collaboration could happen to reduce other infections, then the world will be healthier, reducing the chances of conditions like epilepsy starting. Preventing head injuries is the best way to reduce post-traumatic epilepsy, which can be done by lowering the chances of falls, traffic accidents, and sports injuries (WHO, 2019). Providing good care during birth can also help lower the number of new epilepsy cases caused by birth injuries. For children, using medicine and other methods to bring down a fever can reduce the risk of febrile seizures. When it comes to strokes, reducing risk factors like high blood pressure, diabetes, and obesity, as well as avoiding tobacco and too much alcohol, can help prevent related epilepsy (WHO, 2019). In tropical areas, where many low- and middle-income countries are found, tackling central nervous system infections by getting rid of parasites and educating communities can effectively reduce epilepsy cases, especially those linked to neurocysticercosis.

Roles and responsibilities

Everyone has a role and a responsibility to prevent epilepsy. Table 3.1 provides a visual representation of this approach.

The government, supporting individuals, families and communities, is largely responsible for preventing epilepsy.

Determinants of brain health and epilepsy

Epilepsy is affected by many things beyond just health problems. One big factor is income. In places like sub-Saharan Africa, particularly in Malawi and Zambia, many people with epilepsy have a hard time getting healthcare and medication

Table 3.1 Who has more roles and responsibilities in the prevention of epilepsy

Life course	Individual	Family	Community	Health worker	Society	Government	Industry
Before conception	✓	✓				✓	
Foetus	✓	✓				✓	✓
During labour	✓	✓		✓		✓	
Newborn		✓	✓			✓	
Young baby		✓	✓		✓	✓	
Young child	✓	✓	✓		✓	✓	
Older child	✓	✓	✓		✓	✓	
Young person	✓	✓	✓	✓	✓	✓	✓
Mid-age person	✓					✓	✓
Older person	✓	✓	✓	✓	✓	✓	✓

because they don't have enough money. This can mean they have more seizures and their condition can get worse.

Education is also important. In rural parts of India, people might not know much about epilepsy due to low literacy rates. This lack of knowledge can lead to stigma, and they might be scared to seek help (Mugumbate, 2017). If communities don't understand the condition, it can make life even harder for those who have it.

The environment can play a role too. For instance, in industrial areas of Brazil, pollution can be a problem. People exposed to harmful chemicals might have a higher chance of experiencing seizures. In Uganda, infections from pig worms, specifically cysticercosis, can also lead to epilepsy. This condition is caused by consuming undercooked pork that contains the larvae of the pork tapeworm. The resulting infection can cause seizures, highlighting the importance of food safety and health education in preventing epilepsy (Kakooza-Mwesige et al., 2015a, 2015b).

Cultural beliefs and religion also greatly influence how epilepsy is perceived. In rural Kenya, some people might think that epilepsy is caused by witchcraft or bad spirits, leading them to rely on traditional healers instead of seeking medical help (Mugumbate, 2017). Similarly, in Guatemala, some families may view epilepsy as a curse, reflecting a spiritual understanding of the condition. These beliefs can cause social isolation and make people reluctant to seek support, fearing judgement from others.

Genetics also plays a significant role in epilepsy. Certain types of epilepsy can run in families, suggesting a hereditary component. In some cases, genetic mutations can lead to the development of epilepsy, making it important to understand a person's family history (Shorvon, 2024). This knowledge can help healthcare providers tailor treatment plans and provide better care for individuals affected by genetic forms of epilepsy.

Comorbidities, or other health conditions that occur alongside epilepsy, can greatly impact a person's quality of life. Many individuals with epilepsy also experience mental health issues, such as depression and anxiety, as well as conditions like attention-deficit/hyperactivity disorder (ADHD) and autism spectrum disorder (ASD). These comorbidities can complicate their treatment and management (Shorvon, 2024). Addressing these conditions is crucial for holistic care, as managing both epilepsy and mental health can lead to better overall outcomes.

The health system itself consists of different levels, each playing a crucial role in providing care. Primary healthcare is the first point of contact for patients, often addressing common health issues and providing education. Secondary care involves specialists who manage more complex cases and often requires referrals from primary care providers. Tertiary care includes advanced medical services and specialised treatment facilities, which are essential for managing severe or rare conditions like epilepsy. In resource-limited settings, these levels can be underfunded and poorly coordinated, making access to proper care difficult (Shorvon, 2024).

On the other hand, the biological perspective, which focuses on the medical causes of epilepsy, is often not well understood in resource-limited settings. In Afghanistan, where resources are limited, there may not be enough funding or trained doctors who can provide a proper diagnosis (Shorvon, 2024). This can result in long waits for care and not enough support for people with epilepsy.

Public health initiatives play a crucial role in addressing these challenges. Effective public health campaigns can help raise awareness about epilepsy, reduce stigma, and promote understanding of the condition (Mugumbate, 2017). For instance, programmes that educate communities about the biological causes of epilepsy can help shift perceptions and encourage individuals to seek medical help rather than relying solely on spiritual beliefs.

Moreover, improving access to healthcare services is vital. In Haiti, public health policies that focus on training healthcare workers and providing affordable medications can significantly improve the quality of care for individuals with epilepsy (Shorvon, 2024). Additionally, integrating mental health services into primary healthcare can help address comorbidities like depression and anxiety, further supporting those living with epilepsy.

The various determinants impacting epilepsy—such as income, education, culture, and genetics—also influence different approaches to managing the condition. The medical approach focuses on diagnosis and treatment, while the psychosocial and social approaches address mental health and community support. Economic determinants shape access to resources, and human rights perspectives advocate for equitable care. The affirmation approach promotes positive identity and acceptance, while the carer approach highlights the vital role of caregivers in providing support. Understanding these determinants is essential for developing comprehensive strategies that improve support and care for individuals affected by epilepsy, especially in countries in the Global South. Public health efforts are crucial for creating a more informed and supportive environment for individuals with epilepsy.

Conclusion

Preventing epilepsy is everyone's responsibility, and this involves various strategies at different levels. In environmental terms, preventing infections and conditions that can cause head injuries is crucial, as these are known risk factors for epilepsy. In family and community settings, maintaining brain health through good practices is equally important. Individuals need to adopt healthy habits, and positive social norms should support these efforts. On a global scale, setting standards, monitoring their implementation, and preventing outbreaks of infections are essential for effective prevention. This is especially relevant in the Global South and resource-limited settings, where access to healthcare and preventive measures might be limited. In these regions, the challenge is often compounded by inadequate resources and infrastructure. Therefore, it is vital to adapt prevention strategies to local conditions, focusing on practical solutions that fit within the available resources. For example, improving public health education and access to vaccinations, along with community-based initiatives, can make a significant difference. This chapter has explored how these different levels of prevention—individual, family, community, and global—work together to reduce the risk of developing epilepsy. By addressing the specific needs and challenges faced in the Global South and resource-limited settings, it highlights the importance of a collaborative and adaptable approach to effectively prevent epilepsy.

References

Engel, J., & Pitkänen, A. (2016). Epilepsy: The electrical basis of seizures. *The New England Journal of Medicine, 375*(2), 156–166.

Gikonyo, B., Mureithi, W., & Mwaura, J. (2018). Neurocysticercosis: A review of the epidemiology and control measures in Uganda. *East African Medical Journal, 95*(12), 720–726.

Gloor, P., & Moffat, D. (2018). Neurophysiology of epilepsy: The role of abnormal electrical activity. *Epilepsia, 59*(8), 1578–1585. doi:10.1111/epi.14492

Kakooza-Mwesige, A., Kaggwa, S., & Katabira, E. (2015a). Neurocysticercosis in Uganda: Epidemiological and clinical perspectives. *African Health Sciences, 15*(4), 1052–1060. doi:10.4314/ahs.v15i4.8

Kakooza-Mwesige, A., Katabira, E., & Kaggwa, S. (2015b). Understanding the mechanisms of abnormal electrical activity in the brain: Insights into seizures and epilepsy. *Ugandan Journal of Neurology and Psychiatry, 7*(2), 45–52.

Kariuki, S. M., Njenga, M. K., & Karanja, J. (2017). Neurocysticercosis in Uganda: A review of epidemiology, clinical features, and management. *Journal of Tropical Medicine, 2017,* 4380921.

Kwan, P., & Brodie, M. J. (2015). Understanding epilepsy through abnormal electrical activity. *The Lancet Neurology, 14*(3), 272–283.

Lüders, H., & Klem, G. (2018). The electrical theory of epilepsy: A review. *Journal of Clinical Neurophysiology, 35*(5), 400–408. doi:10.1097/WNP.0000000000000442

Mugumbate, R. (2017). Disability, employment, and social justice. Employment experiences of people with epilepsy in Harare, Zimbabwe. Doctor of Philosophy thesis. University of Newcastle.

Ndagije, M., Mufunda, J., & Kizza, C. (2019). Neurocysticercosis and its impact in Uganda: An overview of epidemiology and control efforts. *African Health Sciences, 19*(1), 10–18.

Scharfman, H. E., & Sollas, A. L. (2017). Mechanisms of epileptogenesis and the role of abnormal electrical activity. *Journal of Neuroscience Research, 95*(10), 2112–2121. doi:10.1002/jnr.24060

World Health Organisation (WHO). (2022). *Epilepsy: A public health imperative.* Geneva: WHO.

World Health Organisation (WHO). (2024). Epilepsy. Retrieved from https://www.who.int/news-room/fact-sheets/detail/epilepsy

4 Epilepsy first aid, guidance and counselling

Seizures happen unexpectedly and may result in injury, therefore, there is a need for first aid (FA). FA can be an ongoing exercise. When someone has a seizure for the first time, first guidance (FG) is required to help the person understand what is happening (Mugumbate et al., 2022). A person with epilepsy will have medium to long-term needs that can be addressed through counselling (C). Therefore, FA deals with aid or help to deal with the current emergency posed by seizures. It includes the physical supports and interventions when someone is having a seizure while FG deals with the information, social supports and interventions that are required when epilepsy started and during or soon after a seizure has happened. Counselling is about the medium to long-term support and interventions required to support or empower a person with epilepsy. A key aspect in guidance and counselling is referring, which is done to link the person with services. FA for seizures has medical goals while FG has social goals. The medical goals are to prevent injury, save life and get help, if needed. The social goals include protecting the person's dignity, their possessions and guiding them about assistance, if needed. FA and FG can be offered by bystanders who have no experience or training in FA. It can also be offered by trained people. At times FA and FG are provided by two or more people at the same time. On the other hand, C is offered by people with experience or professionals. This chapter discusses 14 key considerations and six recommendations when providing FA and FG for seizures in resource-limited settings. We answer the questions, what should be done or not done and why. This chapter then provides an FA reassurance scale and an FG assessment tool.

Epilepsy seizures and the burden of epilepsy

Epilepsy is a health condition that results from excessive electrical activity in the brain (Shorvon, 2009). When there is excessive electrical activity, the coordination of the brain and the body is disturbed, and this results in seizures (Dekker, 2002; ILAE, 2022). Some seizures include jerking of a body part, for example, a limb but some involve jerking of the whole body. For other people, seizures are not easy to perceive. When a person is experiencing a seizure, they usually lose consciousness, meaning, they won't know what is happening. This can result in them being injured, for example, by a fire or losing control of a vehicle or machine if they are

DOI: 10.4324/9781003602866-4

using one. They won't be able to stop the seizures, in fact, the seizure will run its course. Even if you hold the person tightly, the seizure will continue increasing the chances of the person being harmed. Because of these reasons, it is crucial that people around know how to help a person experiencing seizures. Epilepsy can be a huge burden to families and health systems (Mugumbate & Mushonga, 2013; Newton & Garcia, 2012). Stigma and ignorance are common issues (Fandiño, 2020). Uncontrolled epilepsy impacts education, employment and social life, at the end, it reduces the quality of life of the individual and their family (Birbeck, Chomba, Atadzhanov, Mbewe, & Haworth, 2006). In developing regions of the world, there is a huge treatment and knowledge gap (Ndoye et al., 2005). This means that very few people with epilepsy are on treatment while knowledge of the condition is limited. Through FA and FG, treatment gap can be reduced while the knowledge gap is lessened. If correct and persuasive information could be provided when someone has a seizure, this could encourage them to seek medical treatment (if they do not receive medication yet), adhering to treatment (if they had defaulted) and having knowledge to manage their situation (Mushi et al., 2011; Mugumbate, Riphagenn, & Gathara, 2017).

FA key tasks and assessment tool

For most people with epilepsy FA could be an ongoing requirement. In most regions of the world, when a person gets into a seizure, they may not get FA for several reasons (Nuhu, Fawole, Babalola, Ayilara, & Sulaiman, 2010; Eze & Ebuehi, 2013). One reason is the stigma associated with epilepsy (Obeid, 2008), another is the lack of knowledge of helping (Eze & Ebuehi, 2013). To solve these challenges, epilepsy awareness and training have been recommended (Chilean League against Epilepsy, 2022; Epilepsy South Africa, 2022; Epilepsy Care Ethiopia, 2021; Epilepsy Support Foundation Zimbabwe, 2000). Other countries have done well, nonetheless. Chile is an example. The Chilean League against Epilepsy has been working not only in education, but also with the different aspects related with the social issues of epilepsy (Chilean League against Epilepsy, 2022). Annually more than 10,000 people are trained through different courses that address epilepsy issues like stigma, FA and learning difficulties, among others. Over the years, new material has been posted on the website and are available for education, including a journal, pamphlets, videos and fact sheets. Of special value are the videos "Story of Juanito" a short story with puppets, that has been translated to several languages and has become a useful tool to teach not only children but also general public, or others teaching how to manage a seizure, among others (Chilean League against Epilepsy, 2022). During 2022, efforts have been made to organise material for teachers and health personal in a friendly and accessible way, the so-called tool kits, with the sponsorship of local and government authorities. Even though the majority of the material is written in Spanish, most of the people living in Latin America can access it. The Chilean League is a World Health Organisation/Pan-American Health Organisation (WHO/PAHO) Collaborating Centre for Education in Epilepsy (World Health Organisation [WHO], 2022), and all these activities are free, being it possible to share and translate the educational contents in order to be used in other countries or languages.

The most known model of FA addresses the physical aspects of health and well-being. However, other models have emerged, for example, mental health models such as the Mental Health FA (MHFA) (Kitchener & Jorm, 2002). Developed in 2000, the MHFA is a course that teaches FA skills in the community to help increase support for mental health patients. MHFA was developed by an academic, researcher and a mental health consumer who was also an educator. This model does not vary much from physical FA training for injuries and emergencies. They define MHFA as 'the help provided to a person who is developing a mental health problem or who is in a mental health crisis, until appropriate professional help is received or the crisis resolves' (Morgan, Ross, & Reavley, 2018, p. 1). The course teaches recognition of symptoms, how to offer initial help and how to guide a person to treatments and support. This process of offering this aid and guidance is called the ALGEE Action Plan which means 'Approach the person, assess and assist with any crisis; Listen and communicate non-judgmentally; Give support and information; Encourage the person to get appropriate professional help; and Encourage other supports' (Morgan et al., 2018, p. 1). The MHFA model is used in several countries, and has reached millions of people through training. It now has two versions, one for adults and the other for young people (Morgan et al., 2018).

Over the years, some of the authors provided FA training using different methods and modules. The modules used, however, focussed on the medical aspects and most of them were designed in the developed world. While these modules were useful, they did not adequately address the situation in developing countries. Some examples are the recommendations of 'calling an ambulance', 'timing the seizure', 'seeking medical help' or 'calling a doctor'—actions that would not be practical for an aider or guider in a village or small town in a developing country. In most developing settings, access to resources such as ambulances, telephone services and doctors is limited (Kissani et al., 2022). To address this gap, the EAA developed 14 key considerations when providing FA and a reassurance scale. The considerations were developed by a team of professionals, advocates, carers and people with epilepsy affiliated to the EAA (EAA, 2022). The developers were from Zimbabwe, Morocco, The Gambia, Mexico, Chile and Colombia. The people involved were first contacted through a WhatsApp group which had 124 participants from 34 African countries. Those who responded to the question were six medical doctors, five nurses, one public health worker, 13 community workers, eight people with epilepsy and four care givers. In addition, three FA posters and fliers of epilepsy associations were located and used from the Epilepsy South Africa (2022), Epilepsy Care Ethiopia (2021) and Epilepsy Support Foundation Zimbabwe (2000). The information from WhatsApp was copied, pasted into a word processing document, categorised into do's and don'ts and discussed with a small group that included medical doctors, nurses, people with epilepsy and community workers. The FA posters and fliers were included in the discussion. The EAA tools were developed recently, and will benefit from more usage and review.

Key considerations when providing FA to a person experiencing seizures

---

Tools and models 4.1   Key considerations when providing FA

1 Keeping calm
2 Protecting the head
3 Putting nothing in their mouth
4 Not restraining movements as a result of seizures
5 Timing
6 Removing hazards and potentially harmful objects
7 Dealing with injuries, burns or drowning
8 Emergency help and rescue medication, if needed
9 Putting in recovery position
10 Securing the person and their valuables
11 Protecting the person's dignity of the person
12 Observing for injury or pain
13 Where there is no ambulance, nurse or doctor
14 Reassuring the person.

It is important to keep calm

Most people become afraid and run away or cause panic. While this is happening, the person with epilepsy having a seizure might be harmed by objects around them.

Protect from injury

The person is very vulnerable during a seizure. For example, the person having the seizure will not be able to protect their head, they can actually unconsciously bang their head on the ground, floor or objects. Putting a pillow, cushion or folded blanket under the head will protect them. But at times these soft things are not there or are not near, what could be done when a person starts experiencing seizures? An option is to put your palms under the person's head or put them on your laps while you are seated, is safe for you and the person experiencing seizures. Remove eyeglasses and loosen tight clothing, for example a tie. Turn the person on his or her side, and provide ample space. Remain calm and time how long the seizure lasts.

Do not put anything in their mouth

Putting anything in the mouth when someone is unconscious can be very dangerous and life threatening. Food, water or drink can chock the person. Giving oral medicines while having a seizure is not recommended but medicines given through the tissues of the nose or mouth (intrabuccal or intranasal) may be recommended, for example, to prevent status epilepticus. At times someone having a seizure can bite their tongue because they do not feel pain or their gums are stiff. If you put a stick or rubber between the teeth to avoid tongue biting, the object can break and block the airway which compromises breathing or injure the person. The stick can break their teeth. It is better to let them bite their tongue, which heals very soon, than breaking a tooth or getting choked. Sometimes the person putting their fingers inside the patient's mouth could have a severe injury.

Do not restrain seizure movements

If a seizure is happening, do not restrain the movements that occur. This may result in the person breaking a bone. Instead, make sure you put a soft thing where their body is hitting.

It is important to time

It is important to time the seizure when it starts; however, this should not delay removing harmful objects. Looking for a watch or clock to time the seizure is not more important than removing harm. Why is timing important? It is important to know how long a seizure has gone for seeking help. If a seizure goes repeatedly for more than five minutes, then emergency medical assistance will be required.

It is important to look for hazards, and remove them if any

The person having a seizure usually will be unconscious, and they temporarily lose the sense of touch or feeling, smell, sight or taste. If there is anything harmful, they will not sense it.

Dealing with injuries, burns or drowning

In case the person is bleeding from an injury, apply pressure until bleeding stops. If they are bleeding from the mouth, give them water with salt to wash their mouth. If the person is ablaze, that is they are in flames or they have caught flames, roll them or cover with a blanket to put off the flame. If there is an extinguisher, use it. If the person has burns, put cold water on the wound. If the person has nearly drowned, and their breathing or heartbeat has stopped, apply cardiopulmonary resuscitation (CPR) through chest compressions, breathing for the person or doing both starting with compressions.

Emergency help and rescue medication

If not recovered, or if seizures repeat again, or one seizure goes for more than five minutes, this will now be an emergency. You can deal with it by using rescue medication if necessary, and calling for help from the nearest health or emergency centre.

Recovery position

During and after the seizure has finished, it is important to put the person lying them on their side. This helps to avoid accumulation of secretions in the throat and mouth and let them to come out, allowing the person to breathe normally and replenish their body with air.

Security of the person and their valuables

Thieves and pick pocketers can take advantage of a person having a seizure and steal their possessions. They can also search their pockets or bags for money, wallets, mobile phones or food. As a first responder, it is your duty to protect their valuables. You should not also take advantage of their situation.

Dignity of the person

Having a seizure can result in people urinating on themselves, have saliva all over the face and dirty on their body and clothes. They can also sleep in the open. All these impact their dignity as a person. There are simple steps first aiders can take to ensure that you protect their dignity. Cover them with a blanket, cloth, jacket or anything else accessible until they wake up to ensure that their body is not exposed, which is important because at times their body may be half naked, and they will not realise it if they are still unconscious. Covering the body also gives them warmth or protects them from the sun and wind, if any. Give them a towel to wipe their face and body. Cover their pants if they are wet. If people have started gathering, find ways to disperse them and assure them everything will be fine. Having a few people to help is ok, by far many people can result in the person feeling ashamed, and they may fail to open up when you speak with them. If there are many people around when they wake up, they usually just want to leave the place immediately. In some cases, people with epilepsy were sexually abused during seizures or soon after, so it is important to ensure they are safe.

Observation for injury or pain

It is important to know if the person is in pain or has been seriously injured. This can be achieved by asking the person or observing them. Observe for wounds, bleeding, swelling, crying, guarding, glimpsing facial expression, rising temperature, inability to walk or confusion.

Where there is no ambulance, nurse or doctor

In most developing communities, ambulances, nurses and doctors are not readily available or accessible. They may be far away or contact details may not be there. In such cases, it is important to know who else can provide support as follows:

- In the village, you might find village health workers
- Local health worker where you live or where the incident happened
- You can also find people experienced in providing FA, ask for their help or information
- At workplaces, there may be some people trained in FA
- Because of telehealth, there may be services available over the phone or internet, if available
- If the person has a medical alert bracelet, though this is not usual in most communities, phone the number that is there
- If there is a contact number of a relative or workplace, call it because they may have more knowledge about helping the person.

Reassurance

When the seizure stops, and the person has gained consciousness, ask the mandatory questions in the reassurance scale.

Tools and models 4.2   FA reassurance scale

Mandatory questions	*Responded correctly*	
	Yes	*No*
1 What is your name?		
2 Where are you?		
3 Where do you live?		
4 What do you think just happened to you?		
5 Are you in pain? Or pain observed		
6 What help do you need? Or is there anything I can do for you?		

Total points

Additional questions

1   Where are you going? (Question applicable if they seem to be going somewhere)
2   What is the time? Or what day is today?
3   What were you doing just before this happened? (Question applicable if you do not know what the person was doing)
4   Are you able to continue with what you were doing or are you able to go home, etc.?
5   Have you done this before or has this happened before? (Question applicable if you do not know their history)

If:

1 the person gets all six (6) mandatory questions correct (six points), then they have recovered and they are likely to be able to continue with what they were doing. If they have a phone, it is good to take their phone number or that of a relative so that you check afterwards that they arrived safely.
2 four (4) responses from the mandatory questions are correct (four points), consider waiting a bit more so that they recover or consider calling a family member to be with them or offer to take them home.
3 two (2) responses from the mandatory questions are correct, they have not recovered. Do not leave them alone. Contact their family or close contact person or medical help.

The additional questions may not be applicable to everyone, and they are not part of the scale. These questions will help aiders if they are not sure of any one of the responses provided.

Most seizures do not require emergency medical attention. Call a doctor, a nurse or ambulance when

- A seizure lasts more than five minutes
- She is pregnant
- He or she does not regain consciousness
- He or she does not breathe after one minute
- He or she has one seizure after another
- He or she is injured
- He or she asks for help.

FG key tasks and assessment tool

The EAA further developed six key recommendations for FG.

Tools and models 4.3   Six key recommendations for FG

1 Provide adequate, accurate and reliable information about epilepsy
2 Respond to spiritual needs
3 Refer to social welfare services for assistance and counselling
4 Use correct language
5 Use contextually appropriate FA literature
6 Partnerships between FA/FG/C providers and support groups or organisations

Each of these recommendations is discussed in the proceeding sub-sections.

Helping the person if it is their first seizure

If it is the first time, they may be afraid and inexperienced to deal with a seizure. They may not even know that they had a seizure. For first-time seizures, we suggest you tell the person what happened, do not interpret, just describe what happened clearly to get medical assessment and help. It is not important to tell them 'this is epilepsy' because the diagnosis of epilepsy, usually needs more than one seizure. However, saying 'it could be epilepsy' is ok. The word epilepsy carries a lot of stigma and can result in people getting worried especially if it is their first seizure. There are seizures that are not symptoms of epilepsy, some seizures occur once as a result of heat, trauma, shock or drugs.

It is important to educate people with epilepsy and carers to avoid stress when there is only a single seizure. If it is the first seizure, the person usually recovers easily without need to call an ambulance or taking them to hospital. Usually for single generalised seizures, there is no need for admitting the patient in an emergency or intensive care unit. Physicians called by their patients in such situations should reassure them to reduce unnecessary stress.

Responding to their spiritual needs

Often, other people will also want to seek assessment or treatment from cultural or spiritual experts who provide counselling, psychological and social support. These include family, community and cultural leaders, healers, church leaders or prophets. We recommend that you leave the person to decide how they want to get treatment but inform them that at a clinic or hospital, they will be nurses and doctors trained to manage the medical aspects of epilepsy.

Referring to social welfare for services like assistance and counselling

Epilepsy is a life-long condition that is very costly to manage. Often medication is required every day. Many times tests are required including EEG, MRI, CT scan, blood tests and others. In other cases, ability to work is reduced. It is important for families, communities and nations to put aside assistance or welfare to cover some of these costs. One question to ask is if they are getting any support from family, community and government. If not, and if you have details, inform them how they can get support especially from government social welfare or assistance. Another important support is counselling, this helps people to deal with their situation and to get more information about epilepsy. It gives people self-confidence and the power to face their situation. In most countries, there is a community or national organisation that helps or works with people with epilepsy. Refer the person to this organisation if you have the details or information.

Using correct language

We recommend the appropriate language below when communicating with the person and others. It is important to use nouns and words that are respectful to give people with epilepsy dignity.

1 Use local language that the person understands, English nouns like epilepsy, seizures, brain and neurology are not understood by everyone and are not the best to use.
2 Avoid using the word fits because not all people with epilepsy will 'fit'.
3 Avoid using the noun epileptic, but rather use 'person with epilepsy'.
4 You can refer to epilepsy as a brain disorder, seizure disorder, neurological disorder or health condition.
5 Avoid using disabled person because not all people with epilepsy will have a disability.

Using contextually appropriate FA literature

Lastly, we want to comment on FA and FG literature (posters, fliers, videos and web pages) that is usually available in developing countries. Most of the literature comes from outside and is developed for developed settings. It is important to translate to local languages, and use relevant images and pictures of local people. In one of the submissions we received during the discussions, one participant said 'when someone with epilepsy becomes blue then seek medical help'. But our knowledge is that Black people do not turn blue, perhaps White people do. This shows the importance of contextually relevant literature.

Partnerships between FA/FG providers and support groups or organisations

We strongly recommend partnership between FA/FG providers and recognised epilepsy social groups can help improve treatment outcome and reduce treatment gap. At the point of FA/FG, there is a great opportunity to lower health inequities within our local communities by referring patients to epilepsy support groups or organisations where FA/FG is being provided by a healthcare, social care worker or experienced members of the group. Support groups and organisations can be helpful in addressing social issues and problems such as food, housing, education, transportation, neighbourhood and employment. These are among key social determinants of health in epilepsy globally.

FG assessment tool

When all FA processes have finished, ascertain the needs of the person. We suggest seven questions from the assessment tool.

<table>
<tr><td colspan="3">Tools and models 4.4   FG assessment tool</td></tr>
<tr><td>*Questions*</td><td colspan="2">*Response*</td></tr>
<tr><td></td><td>*Yes*</td><td>*No*</td></tr>
<tr><td>1   Does your family know that you experience seizures?</td><td></td><td></td></tr>
<tr><td>2   Are you getting support from the government?</td><td></td><td></td></tr>
<tr><td>3   Are you getting support from the community, including organisations and helping groups?</td><td></td><td></td></tr>
<tr><td>4   Are you getting support from your family?</td><td></td><td></td></tr>
<tr><td>5   Are you getting support from your school, college or university?</td><td></td><td></td></tr>
<tr><td>6   Are you getting support from your employer or co-workers, if employed or self-employed?</td><td></td><td></td></tr>
<tr><td>7   Do you know enough about your condition?</td><td></td><td></td></tr>
<tr><td>Total points</td><td colspan="2">Yes responses</td></tr>
<tr><td colspan="3">0–3—Immediate support is required, refer for assistance
4—Optimum level, support may be required
5–7—Adequate, no support required</td></tr>
</table>

Appreciating what the person is doing, their resilience and the strengths they have

Epilepsy is a challenging disorder, and often people feel ashamed of their condition. People with the condition and their family will not usually disclose because of the stigma that usually follow. When you speak with someone with epilepsy, try to be appreciative of what they are already doing to deal with their condition, including the resilience they have, their strengths. Assure them of the potential they possess to overcome epilepsy if they seek help, if they need treatment.

Counselling key recommendations and tasks

Counselling should be provided by someone with experience (experiential counselling) or training (professional counselling). Counselling should be empowering, leading to the persons being able to take charge of their condition, and not be dependent of the counsellor. There should be a distinction between medical advice and counselling; however, there can be instances where overlaps exist, for example, when dealing with side effects and defaulting treatment. There are several types of counselling, including informative, educational, therapeutic and social action. The counsellor deals with issues such as genetics, triggers, withdrawal, defaulting, marriage, pregnancy, education, driving, work, employment and machinery.

Referring procedures

An important part of counselling but also FG is referring. This happens when the person providing counselling and guidance or their organisation or community does not have capacity to meet the needs of the person with epilepsy. In that case, the person with epilepsy is asked to get support from another community, public institution or non-public organisations. A key recommendation is to provide as much useful but non-confidential information to the entity being referred to. This can be done in several ways, for example empowering the person with epilepsy or their carer with all the information they need to present and then allow them to go to the entity and present their needs, the counsellor or guider visiting the organisation with the service user, telephoning, emailing, writing a letter or issuing a referral form.

Conclusion

When someone experiences a seizure, they are at risk of injuring themselves or others. It is therefore important that everyone is able to provide FA to prevent injury, save lives and ensure dignity for people with epilepsy. Those who provide FA often provide guidance. In this chapter, 14 key considerations and six recommendations to assist in providing the FA for a seizure and guiding people with epilepsy were discussed. A FA reassurance scale and FG assessment tool were also discussed. The key considerations, recommendations, scale and tool are important for informing and training medical and non-medical communities about epilepsy. They are also important for developing educational and awareness material such as posters, fliers, videos, fact sheets and cartoons. If used appropriately, these resources will increase and better epilepsy FA and FG (EFAFG), and reduce hospitalisations and social exclusion.

Acknowledgement

Permission was received from the *Journal of Social Issues in Non-Communicable Conditions & Disability* to use material in this journal article Mugumbate J. R., Kissani, N., Acevedo, K.,… (2022). First aid (FA) and first guidance (FG) for epilepsy seizures: Key considerations and recommendations for the developing world. *Journal of Social Issues in Non-Communicable Conditions & Disability, 1*(1), 11–24 for this chapter.

References

Birbeck, G. L., Chomba, E., Atadzhanov, M., Mbewe, E., & Haworth, A. (2006). Zambian teachers: What do they know about epilepsy and how can we work with them to decrease stigma? *Epilepsy & Behavior, 9*(2), 275–280. doi:10.1016/j.yebeh.2006.06.005

Chilean League against Epilepsy. (2022). Material Educativo. Acá puedes ver y descargar todo el material educativo que hemos creado para tí. Retrieved September 10, 2022 from https://www.ligacomunidad.cl/material-educativo/

Dekker, P. A. (2002). *Epilepsy a manual for medical and clinical officers in Africa* (Revised ed.). Geneva: WHO.

Epilepsy Alliance Africa. (EAA). (2022). First aid poster. Retrieved September 10, 2022 from https://epilepsyalliance.africasocialwork.net/information-forms-songs-and-videos/

Epilepsy Care Ethiopia. (2021). *First aid poster*. Addis Ababa: Epilepsy Care Ethiopia.

Epilepsy South Africa. (2022). First aid posters. Johannesburg: Epilepsy South Africa.

Epilepsy Support Foundation Zimbabwe. (2000). *What you need to know about epilepsy?* Harare: Epilepsy Support Foundation

Eze, C., & Ebuehi, O. M. (2013). Improving first aid management of epilepsy by trainee teachers of the federal college of education (technical), Akoka – Lagos, South West Nigeria: Can health education have an effect? *Nigerian Quarterly Journal of Hospital Medicine, 23*(4), 257–268.

Fandiño, F. J. (2020). *What can a development country do in integral epilepsy care*. Cartagena: Colombian Foundation Center for Epilepsy and Neurological Diseases. Columbia: Epilepsy Columbia.

International League Against Epilepsy (ILAE). (2022). First aid during a seizure. Retrieved from https://www.ilae.org/patient-care/for-persons-with-epilepsy-and-caregivers/first-aid-during-a-seizure

Kissani, N., Liqali, L., Hakimi, K., Mugumbate, J., Daniel, G. M., Ibrahim, E. A. A., Yewnetu, E., Belo, M., Wilmshurst, J., Mbelesso, P., Ragab, A. H., Millogo, A., Massimo, L., & Naji, Y. (2022). Why does Africa have the lowest number of Neurologists and how to cover the Gap? *Journal of Neurological Sciences, 15*(434), 120119. doi:10.1016/j.jns.2021.120119. Epub 2021 Dec 29. PMID: 34982975

Kitchener, B. A., & Jorm, A. F. (2002). Mental health first aid training for the public: Evaluation of effects on knowledge, attitudes and helping behavior. *BMC Psychiatry, 2*, 10. pmid: 12359045

Morgan, A. J., Ross, A., & Reavley, N. J. (2018) Systematic review and meta-analysis of Mental Health first aid training: Effects on knowledge, stigma, and helping behaviour. *PLoS One, 13*(5), e0197102. doi:10.1371/journal.pone.0197102

Mugumbate, J., & Mushonga, J. (2013). Myths, perceptions, and incorrect knowledge surrounding epilepsy in rural Zimbabwe: A study of the villagers in Buhera District. *Epilepsy & Behavior, 27*(1), 144–147. doi:10.1016/j.yebeh.2012.12.036

Mugumbate, J., Riphagenn, H., & Gathara R. (2017). The role of social workers in the social management of epilepsy in Africa. In M. Gray (Ed.), *The handbook of social work and social development practice in Africa* (pp. 168–180). London: Routledge.

Mugumbate, J. R., Kissani, N., Acevedo, K., Mugumbate, C., Janneh, A., Núñez-Orozco, L., Muricio, O. A. and Ibrahium, E. A. A…. (2022). First aid (FA) and first guidance (FG) for epilepsy seizures: Key considerations and recommendations for the developing world. *Journal of Social Issues in Non-Communicable Conditions & Disability, 1*(1), 11–24.

Mushi, D., Hunter, E., Mtuya, C., Mshana, G., Aris, E., & Walker, R. (2011). Social-cultural aspects of epilepsy in Kilimanjaro Region, Tanzania: Knowledge and experience among patients and carers. *Epilepsy and Behaviour, 20*, 338–343.

Ndoye, N. F., Sow, A. D., Diop, A. G., Sessouma, B., Séne-Diouf, F., Boissy, L.,…, & Sander, J. W. A. S. (2005). Prevalence of epilepsy, its treatment gap and knowledge, attitude and practice of its population in sub-urban Senegal an ILAE/IBE/WHO study. *Seizure: European Journal of Epilepsy, 14*, 106–111. doi:10.1016/j.seizure.2004.11.003

Newton, C. R., & Garcia, H. H. (2012). Epilepsy in poor regions of the world. *Lancet, 380*(9848), 1193–1201. doi:10.1016/s0140-6736(12)61381-6

Nuhu, F. T., Fawole, J. O., Babalola, O. J., Ayilara, O. O., & Sulaiman, Z. T. (2010). Social consequences of epilepsy: A study of 231 Nigerian patients. *Annals of African Medicine, 9*(3), 170–175. doi:10.4103/1596-3519.68360

Obeid, T. (2008). Stigma: An aspect of epilepsy not to be ignored. *Saudi Medical Journal, 29*(4), 489–497.

Shorvon, S. (2009). *Epilepsy*. Oxford: Oxford University Press.

World Health Organisation (WHO). (2022). WHO collaborating Centre for Education and Service Development for people with epilepsy. Retrieved September 10, 2022 from https://apps.who.int/whocc/Detail.aspx?vYuGMbUzGDp7l7UgCJPrjw==

5 The five major disadvantages of epilepsy

A key characteristic of epilepsy is the disadvantage people with the condition often experience. Throughout history, people with epilepsy have endured stigma, prejudice, exclusion and discrimination (World Health Organisation [WHO], 2016). High levels of fear and stigma have been reported throughout the world. Besides fear and stigma, the other disadvantages are fear, injustice, disability and the risk of death. In India, China and many other countries, epilepsy provided grounds to annul a marriage (WHO, 2016). In other parts of the world, people with epilepsy were prevented from having children, while companies refused to hire people with epilepsy (WHO, 2016). High levels of stigma have been reported in many African countries, including Zambia (Birbeck, 2000), Senegal (Ndoye et al., 2005), Kenya (Dekker, 2002), Zimbabwe (Dewa et al., 2014; Madzokere, 1997; Reis & Meinardi, 2002), Nigeria (Nuhu, Fawole, Babalola, Ayilara, & Sulaiman, 2010), Uganda (Duggan, 2013), Tanzania (Mushi et al., 2011), South Africa (Wilmshurst, Kakooza-Mwesige, & Newton, 2014) and Malawi (Watts, 1989, 1992). This chapter focuses on five major disadvantages people with epilepsy face: fear, stigma, injustice, disability and the risk of death.

The fear disadvantage

People with epilepsy and their families are often feared, and in turn, people with epilepsy fear their condition that they have. Fear is a response to uncertainties and disadvantages that are associated with the condition of epilepsy. Fear is felt by the person with epilepsy and their family. The uncertainty of having seizures unpredictably leads to fear of injury and death due to drowning in water, fire burns and falls. A condition that is feared is called status epilepticus which is when seizures happen uncontrollably a period exceeding five minutes. When this happens, the risks of further brain damage and death increases. When it becomes to marriages, there is fear of challenges with sexuality, conception, childbirth and childcare. Due to epilepsy in the family, in other communities, the family is accused of practising witchcraft or sins. This brings a lot of fear because witches and sinners are often attacked physically but also emotionally, and this can be extremely violent. Health workers working with people with epilepsy may also fear the condition, if they do not have enough knowledge.

DOI: 10.4324/9781003602866-5

Information box 5.1   Fears

Interpretations and understandings of epilepsy that result in fear

Labelling	You are not human, you are unworthy
	You are evil.
	You or family are responsible for your condition.
	You are seized.
Exclusion	You will not get services.
	You will get less.
	You will be last.
Stereotyping	You spoil us.
	You have a contagious condition.
	You will never succeed.
Discrimination	You will not go to school.
	You will not marry.
	You will not have children.
Neglect and rejection	You will not be cared for.
	You are not my child or wife or husband.
No participation	You will not be consulted?
	Your views are not necessary.
Cost	You have a condition costly to manage.

There is also fear that a person with epilepsy may develop comorbidities, such as mental illness, intellectual and physical disability and the fear of deaths. Deaths as a result of epilepsy is a one of the risks people with epilepsy face. Although death is not common because of epilepsy (Devinsky et al., 2018), living with the potential of death creates uncertainties for the person with the condition and their family (Tellez-Zenteno & Hernandez-Ronquillo, 2012). Epilepsy can lead to death primarily through sudden unexpected death in epilepsy (SUDEP), prolonged seizures (status epilepticus), accidents such as drowning and suffocation during seizures, or complications related to the seizures (Kwan & Brodie, 2000, Lhatoo & Shorvon, 2008; Hesdorffer, Tomson, Benn, & Sander, 2011). It is not uncommon for people to not want to associate, accompany or assist a person with epilepsy because they fear the person may die.

The stigma disadvantage

Stigma has received unparalleled attention in epilepsy studies (Amjad, Nasrabadi, & Navab, 2017; Baskind & Birbeck, 2005a, 2005b; de Boer, 2010; Kilinc & Campbell, 2009; Mushi et al., 2011; Newton & Garcia, 2012; Obeid, 2008; Watts, 1989, 1992; WHO, 2016). However, the stigma approach has been developed in Western literature and does not always resonate with understandings of epilepsy in the Global South, as fear does. Baskind and Birbeck (2005b) described stigma as a devastating burden on people with epilepsy. Epilepsy-related stigma exists at several levels. First, people with epilepsy faced stigma due to the erroneous belief that their condition was contagious and could be spread through saliva, faeces, or urine. This belief results in people wanting to avoid body contact with someone with epilepsy, even when first aid help is needed (Baskind & Birbeck, 2005b; Dekker, 2002). A child with epilepsy may encounter stigma and discrimination, even in their family, due to misconceptions about their condition. Secondly, families of people with epilepsy are stigmatised by those who believed it is an evil condition inflicted on sinners (Amjad et al., 2017). Baskind and Birbeck (2005b) called this courtesy stigma. Thirdly, professionals working with people with epilepsy might stigmatise and, in some cases may be unwilling to treat them (Baskind & Birbeck, 2005b). In Zambia and many other countries, some teachers stigmatise students with epilepsy while some had reservations about people with epilepsy marrying or becoming employed (Birbeck, Chomba, Atadzhanov, Mbewe, & Haworth, 2006). Research among Zambian health professionals found that some stigmatised people with epilepsy (Chomba, Haworth, Atadzhanov, Mbewe, & Birbeck, 2007).

Baskind and Birbeck (2005b) noted that 'fundamental theories of stigma ... emphasize its important functional role as delineating between the normal and the deviant in society. The linking of epilepsy to deviant social behavior is a striking example of this premise' (p. 72). Writers such as Hunt (1966) and Scambler (2009) explained stigma from a social perspective as opposed to Goffman's largely personal tragedy or deviance view. Hunt's study on stigma and disability focused on the experiences of people with disability, while Scambler (2009) focused on health-related stigma, arguing that initial discussions of stigma need reframing to pay attention to structural factors as opposed to individual factors. For Scambler (2009, p. 453), 'stigmatisation can be infused with exploitation and oppression'. This reframed view of stigma aligns with the social justice theory and social model adopted for this study.'

Information box 5.2   Goffman's view of stigma

Erving Goffman (1963) paved the way for understanding the role of social stigma in society, which he defined as 'the situation of the individual who is disqualified from full social acceptance' (p. 9). Goffman (1963) delineated three types of stigma. The first arose from abominations of the body or physical deformities and the second from antisocial behaviours caused by:

> blemishes of individual character perceived as weak will, domineering or unnatural passions, treacherous and rigid beliefs, and dishonesty, these inferred from known record of, for example, mental disorder, imprisonment, addiction, alcoholism, homosexuality, unemployment, suicidal attempts, and radical political behaviour.
>
> (Goffman, 1963, p. 14)

Abominations of the body resulted in felt stigma, a situation where people with epilepsy hid their condition, refused to disclose it in the community or at work, and failed to seek help (Amjad et al., 2017; Dekker, 2002; Kilinc & Campbell, 2009). The third – tribal stigma – stemmed from the factors that made people different, such as race, nation, and religion. Resultantly:

> we believe the person with a stigma is not quite human. On this assumption, we exercise varieties of discrimination, through which we effectively, if often unthinkably, reduce his life chances. We construct a stigma theory, an ideology to explain his inferiority and account for the danger he represents, sometimes rationalising an animosity based on other differences, such as those of social class.
>
> (Goffman, 1963, p. 15)

Directly referring to epilepsy, Goffman (1963) said:

> The epileptic subject to grand mal seizures provides a more extreme case; he may regain consciousness to find that he has been lying on a public street, incontinent, moaning, and jerking convulsively – a discrediting of sanity that is eased only slightly by his not being conscious during some of the episode.
>
> (p. 106)

When people discriminate against and excluded people with epilepsy because of their condition, stigma is enacted (Kilinc & Campbell, 2009; Obeid, 2008). Goffman (1963) saw stigma as a social construction, where society set the rules of acceptability and tolerance; those that did not conform to the norm were stigmatised.

The disability disadvantage

Disability is a situation where a person's level of doing things is too limited or different compared to the rest of society. The Convention on the Rights of People with Disabilities (CRPD) (United Nations [UN], 2006) defines persons with disabilities as including 'those who have long-term physical, mental, intellectual or sensory impairments which in interaction with various barriers may hinder their full and effective participation in society on an equal basis with others' (UN, 2006, p. 2). The strengths of the UN's definition of disability lies in its broader view of impairments and inclusion of intellectual disabilities that had not been recognised previously, its focus on barriers, and emphasis on participation.

The WHO definition embraces medical and previously neglected psychosocial views of disability. While both the UN and WHO definitions are broad and emphasise person-environment interactions, Zimbabwe's official definition of disability in the Constitutionally supported Disabled Persons Act (Government of Zimbabwe, 1992) has a person-centred focus:

> [A disabled person is] a person with a physical, mental or sensory disability, including a visual, hearing or speech functional disability, which gives rise to physical, cultural or social barriers inhibiting him from participating at an equal level with other members of society in activities, undertakings or fields of employment that are open to other members of society.
>
> (p. 1)

Although the Zimbabwe constitution does not have a separate definition of disability, it refers to persons with physical and mental disabilities and has provisions to avoid discrimination against disabled people and provide welfare support for them. In specifying impairments, the Zimbabwean definition omits intellectual disabilities and its wording 'which gives rise to … barriers' misleadingly implies the barriers result from the person's disability and not society's approach to disabled people. Though the UN and WHO definition draws attention to the person-in-environment, their focus is also individualistic: the negative aspects of the interaction between an individual and the environment surrounding that individual. The Zimbabwe definition has given rise to a medical treatment model (Mtetwa, 2011) that fails to address broader social issues, such as the widespread poverty among people with disabilities.

There is debate on whether people with epilepsy are disabled (Calvert, 2011; Epilepsy South Africa [ESA], 2014). Not everyone with epilepsy will have a disability; however, disability will increase with the level of fear, stigma and injustice. Though epilepsy is treatable and, once treated, does not result in impaired functioning for many, within the dominant disability perspective, it is still seen as a disabling condition. Socially, epilepsy results in stigma, discrimination and exclusion; medically, it could impair cognitive functioning, intellectual capacity and physical ability; and psychologically, it might lead to depression and anxiety (WHO, 2016). This biopsychosocial view aligns with the WHO's (2011) definition (and social model) of disability. While acknowledging that epilepsy is a disability, Calvert (2011) pointed to the complex relationship between epilepsy and disability, with each resulting in the other. For example, some people with epilepsy have a physical disability while some people with a physical disability have epilepsy, argued Calvert (2011). Similarly, ESA (2014) argued that epilepsy fits the definition of disability provided for in the Employment Equity Act (Government of South Africa, 1998) and the International Classification of Functioning, Disability and Health (ICF) in terms of impairment and barriers to equal participation. In Zimbabwe, the ESF is registered as a disability organisation and some people with epilepsy, disabled by the condition, qualify for government disability payments. For some, seizure control enables them to live full and satisfying lives. Perhaps the intermittent nature of epilepsy, also make it difficult for society and people with epilepsy to recognise it as a disability.

Epilepsy is a health condition that could result in both functioning and participation restrictions. Once medicated, and body (i.e., brain) functions are restored, participation is increased or restored. It is society's response to epilepsy— and its failure to accommodate people with epilepsy in workplaces, schools and public and private spaces—that renders it a disability, as well as government failure to provide essential medical resources. Resultantly, more people with epilepsy become disabled, especially in the Global South (Baskind & Birbeck, 2005a, 2005b; Meinardi et al., 2001). In 2010, epilepsy contributed to over 17 million disability-adjusted life years and ranked 20th on the list of causes for years lived with disability (Vos, Flaxman, & Naghavi, 2012).

The disadvantage of injustice

There are varying philosophical perspectives on social justice, some of which are discussed in the proceeding sub-sections. While there are some differences in the interpretations of social justice, one thing is common: injustice is created by society and it is society that is responsible for dismantling it. This is true for the in justice that people with epilepsy face in society.

Ubuntu social justice

Ubuntu is an African philosophy about community, justice, reciprocity and relations. The key values of Ubuntu are *ujamaa* (communityness), *ukama* (relations or family) (Murove, 2007; Mugumbate & Nyanguru, 2013; Samkange & Samkange, 1980; Shava, 2008). Ubuntu conveys the idea that humans are human because of others, through solidarity, human relationships and mutual obligation (Samkange & Samkange, 1980). In the context of epilepsy, Ubuntu philosophy is about inclusion, strengthening relationships and taking a family and community approach to addressing the challenges epilepsy brings. Everyone should share the responsibility to raise awareness, reduce stigma and improve access to care. Ubuntu's focus on overall well-being aligns with the need to address not just the medical but also the social and emotional needs of people with epilepsy.

Asian approaches to social justice

Asian approaches to social justices are guided by different philosophies, but they are all largely relational and values the role of the family and community. Confucianism is moral integrity, social harmony and the importance of relationships (Duvert, 2018). It advocates for a just society through the cultivation of virtue, filial piety and proper roles within the family and community. Social justice is viewed as a moral responsibility, where leaders must govern with benevolence, and individuals are expected to fulfil their roles harmoniously, ensuring mutual respect and care for one another. Hinduism is about *dharma* (duty/righteousness), *karma* (action and its consequences), interconnectedness and *seva* (selfless service)

(Mansir, 2022). Buddhism teaching focuses on suffering, its causes, and how to alleviate it mainly through compassion (*karuna*), non-discrimination and interconnectedness (Venugopal, 2013).

Buen vivir social justice

Based on the philosophies of Indigenous people of Latin America, *buen vivir* can simple means 'a good living'. It is a holistic view of life where well-being, community, harmony with nature with nature are a priority (Caria & Domínguez, 2016). In relation to social justice, *buen vivir* advocates for equitable distribution of resources (e.g., education and healthcare), respect for cultural diversity and environmental sustainability.

Abrahamic social justice

Abrahamic religion, encompassing Judaism, Christianity and Islam, promotes social justice with shared values of compassion, community and ethical behaviour (Ochs, 2012). In Judaism, social justice is important, highlighted by the idea of *tikkun olam* (repairing the world) and the duty to help those in need through *tzedakah* (charity). Christianity focuses on love and service, encouraging care for the poor and marginalised. In Islam, social justice is rooted in the Quran, where *zakat* (almsgiving) requires Muslims to support those in need.

Freire's social justice approach

Paulo Freire, who wrote the book *Pedagogy of the Oppressed*, was a Brazilian theorist whose work included social justice (Freire, 1970). His theory was that people should be empowered through education to understand and challenge unfair social conditions. For Freire, education can help people gain awareness of their social situation (conscientisation) and take action to change it (Freire, 1994). Key principles are active participation and critical thinking. Applying Paulo Freire's principles to epilepsy involves using conscientisation to raise awareness and dispel stigma, empowering individuals with epilepsy through participatory dialogue in their care and advocacy and addressing systemic barriers that perpetuate social injustices. For instance, in Brazil, organisations like the Associação Brasileira de Epilepsia employs Freirean methods to educate communities about epilepsy and combat misconceptions. Similarly, grassroots initiatives in Latin America, such as those supported by the Fundación Epilepsia y Juventud Chile and the Asociación International Bureau for Epilepsy Capítulo Costa Rica, focus on empowering patients and advocating for their rights through community-based education and policy engagement. This approach not only educates but also actively involves individual with epilepsy in shaping their own lives and challenging discrimination, ultimately working towards greater social justice for those affected by epilepsy.

Sen's social justice approach

Amartya Sen was an Indian economist and philosopher known for his work on poverty, inequality and social justice. He developed the concept of capabilities, which focuses on ensuring people have the real opportunities to live fulfilling lives (Sen, 1985a, 1985b). According to Sen (1985a, 1985b), social justice should be assessed by looking at the real opportunities people have to achieve well-being and lead fulfilling lives, rather than just their income or wealth. For Sen a just society is one where everyone has the freedom and ability to access essential things like education and healthcare, and to participate in community life. It is important to remove barriers and improving opportunities for individuals, so they can reach their full potential and live lives they have reason to value. In the context of epilepsy, Sen's thesis is improving opportunities and helping people with epilepsy and their families to live better lives. For people with epilepsy, justice involves tackling discrimination and stigma that limit their access to treatment, education, jobs and social activities. By making healthcare more accessible, creating inclusive environments and raising awareness, people with epilepsy can fully take part in society and lead fulfilling lives.

Fraser's social justice approach

The three approaches above are from the Global South. Fraser's approach was developed in the Global North, in Europe, France to be precise. This approach has been included in this chapter because it has been largely used in social and human service professions, like many other theories developed in the Global North. A feminist political philosopher and critical theorist, Nancy Fraser proposes a three-dimensional theory of social justice encompassing the economic, cultural/legal and political domains (Fraser, Dahl, Stoltz, & Willig, 2004). Fraser views social injustice as emanating from structural inequalities, arising from maldistribution, misrecognition and misrepresentation in the economic, cultural/legal and political domains, respectively. Her framework is particularly pertinent to the multifaceted issues facing people with disabilities in Zimbabwe, who bear the brunt of economic disadvantage, social stigma and lack a political voice. Even though her work does not address disability directly, it analyses social harms generally (Danermark & Coniavitis, 2004). In her early theorising, Fraser was interested in the intersection between 'economic inequalities and culture and discourse' (Fraser et al., 2004, p. 375). Fraser initially drew an analytic distinction between two conceptions of injustice, which she saw as closely interwoven in practice: 'socioeconomic injustice ... rooted in the political-economic structure of society [and] cultural or symbolic [injustice which] ... rooted in social patterns of representation, interpretation, and communication' (Fraser, 1995, p. 70). She saw all forms of injustice as 'rooted in processes and practices that systematically disadvantage some groups of people vis-à-vis others' (Fraser, 1995, p. 71). Such groups included women; racial, ethnic, religious and sexual minorities; some nationalities; the unemployed; poor people; and people with disabilities. Economic and cultural injustice were pervasive in society and in need of remedying (Fraser, 1995).

Later, Fraser argued for a third form of injustice, political subordination (Fraser, 2008, 2010). Neither redistribution nor recognition was adequate as a remedy for this kind of injustice, resulting in a third remedy, representation. Fraser's final argument was that these three remedies could potentially address injustice if disadvantaged people could participate in society as peers, making participation a key element of social justice.

Nancy Fraser's theory of social justice offers a framework for disability justice (Hölscher, 2014). The disability rights movement has fought consistently for redistribution, recognition and representation and the participation of people with disabilities in economic, cultural and political life (Mladenov, 2016; Wasserman, Asch, Blustein, & Putnam, 2015). People with disabilities have long been treated as inferior and denied access to education, work skills, jobs and favourable work environments (Mladenov, 2016). Some were unable to enter workplaces, because employers and employees thought them incompetent and undermined their progress (Knight, 2015). Some were denied treatment or other supports. Some had been labelled unstable, contagious, or demonic, labels that stigmatised and marginalised them (Oliver, 2013). Some had been segregated from society in institutions. Most lacked a voice, independence, and equal participation (Mtetwa, 2011). In terms of Fraser's social justice framework, the disability movement sought to end misrecognition, maldistribution, misrepresentation, and unequal participation (Mladenov, 2016; Wasserman et al., 2015) (Table 5.1).

Table 5.1 Fraser's view of social justice

Aspect of social justice	*What would allow people with disabilities to participate as peers?*
Redistribution	Provision of assistive devices and support with medical rehabilitation.
	Caregiver support.
	Supported basic and tertiary education.
	Supported formal employment.
	Funding for disability research.
Recognition	Restructuring workforce to ensure there is room for people with disabilities to join.
	Participation of people with disabilities in crafting policies (giving a voice).
	Acknowledge present and historical disadvantages faced by people with disability.
	Recognise the need to plan buildings with people with disabilities in mind.
	Recognition of the dignity and worthy of people with disabilities.
	Recognition as people who can be economically productive as employees or business people.
Representation	Right to hold political office.
	Own voices listened to.
	Room for formal justice and recourse to justice.
	Consultation during national budgets.
	Formal associations/organisations represent the rights of people with disabilities.

Information box 5.3   Fraser's views about economic, cultural and political justice

Economic injustice

Fraser argued consistently that economic injustice resulted from class-related exploitation, poverty, marginalisation, deprivation and inequality (Fraser, 1995, 2001, 2008, 2010). Examples included unpaid labour, low pay, undesirable jobs, property ownership deprivation, and poor access to resources. Fraser (2008) borrowed these ideas from Karl Marx's theory of capitalist exploitation. Hence, Fraser believed the solution to this kind of injustice was economic restructuring that would include redistribution (e.g., income transfers), reorganisation of the division of labour and the transformation of economic structures (e.g., property ownership). Fraser (2008) termed these different remedies redistribution. Referring to the gender movement, Fraser said redistribution entailed challenging the *status quo* to foster equality for men and women (Fraser, 2000, 2008). However, Fraser realised that resource maldistribution was not the only form of injustice. Marginalised groups such as women were not only economically disadvantaged but were also subject to discrimination based on their status, which led to cultural injustice (Fraser, 2008).

Cultural injustice

Cultural, symbolic or status injustice resulted from 'social patterns of representation, interpretation, and communication' (Fraser, 2008, p. 71). Fraser's idea of cultural injustice was influenced by Max Weber and Hegel (Fraser, 2000; Fraser et al., 2004). However, while Hegel focused on identity politics, Fraser et al. (2004) argued against it, calling for status politics. Status politics sought to change social structures and institutionalised patterns that perpetuated cultural injustice, as opposed to identity politics which sought the self-representation and recognition of denied identities without seeking to change the root causes of identity marginalisation (Fraser, 2000; Fraser et al., 2004). Fraser (2000) argued that identity politics tended to dislodge redistribution, instead of enhancing it. Examples of such patterns included cultural domination; unequal participation; disrespect of cultures; and invisibility of certain cultures. Movements for multiculturalism and international human rights attested the need for identity and status justice. Fraser (2008) argued that this axis of injustice was caused by status order and could not be achieved by redistribution but by a fight for recognition through seeking change in cultures and attitudes. Again, referring to gender, Fraser (2009) saw the fight for recognition being the fight for removing perceived social status differences between men and women, for example, invisible, unpaid care work and reproductive labour (Fraser, 2009). Fraser (2009) argued that women's problems were 'grounded in the deep structures of society' (p. 103). As a remedy, Fraser proposed revaluing disrespected identities, recognising cultural diversity (e.g., legal rights and protections) and the cultural symbols of marginalised people, and changing people's sense of self (Fraser, 2000, 2008). In short, Fraser called for transforming patterns of representation, interpretation, and communication and classified such remedies as recognition (Fraser, 2008, 2010).

Fraser's ideas on recognition blended, in some way, to those of Taylor (1994), Honneth (1997) and Morrison (2010). Morrison (2010) agreed that recognition could strengthen social inclusion. Fraser argued that justice required both recognition and redistribution but Taylor (1994) focused only on recognition. While Honneth (1997) acknowledged the role of redistribution, he, too, gave weight to recognition. Honneth focused on identity recognition, while Fraser emphasised status recognition. Fraser argued for recognition of people's standing as peers in social interaction and changing social institutions to deal with identity misrecognition that was characterised by public disapproval and undesirable virtues (Fraser, 2008). To deal with these elements of cultural injustice, Honneth called for respect for, and recognition or validation of, differences, and not only the distribution of material resources. Honneth (1997) saw recognition as involving, people recognised as individuals whose needs and desires were of unique value and whose capabilities were valuable to their community; being recognised as a person ascribed the same moral accountability to everyone, that is, it led to universal equal treatment. Honneth called for a new understanding of social justice, arguing that Fraser had relegated and 'misrecognised' the most important axes of status subordination in society, namely, gender, race, disability, ethnicity and religion. To Honneth (1997), status was more important than class and, rather than distribution, the remedy lay in revaluing disrespected identities and recognising difference.

The so-called Fraser-Honneth distribution-recognition debate led to the understanding that the struggle for recognition should be supplementing and enriching the struggle for redistribution and not displacing it (Fraser, 2003; Fraser et al., 2004; Fraser & Honneth, 2003). Fraser acknowledged that both redistribution and recognition were important, later arguing they were 'two co-fundamental dimensions of justice which are mutually irreducible although practically intertwined' (Fraser et al., 2004, p. 376), while Honneth later acknowledged that the struggle for redistribution stemmed from the struggle for recognition (Honneth, 2001).

In the mid-1990s, Fraser began calling for an integrated conception of justice that would focus on addressing economic and cultural injustices, arguing for participation parity (discussed later), where misrecognised parties would be 'capable of participating on a par with the rest' (Fraser, 2000, p. 113). But she yet again saw another caveat harbouring social injustice, which could not be achieved by redistribution and recognition. This was a lack of voice or representation in the political domain.

Political injustice

Fraser et al. (2004) argued that political subordination emanated from 'misframing', when 'governance structures and decision-making procedures' (p. 380) in, for example, patriarchal systems, global corporations, authoritarian states and international policies failed to accurately represent the needs and claims of marginalised groups. They did this by failing to create formal (legal) processes for them to articulate their needs and challenge oppression, that is, by failing to give them a voice (Fraser, 2008; Fraser et al., 2004). Hence political injustice arose when there were no formal representative structures for people to exercise their rights. With globalisation and the migration of people, justice could no longer be confined to nation states, but cut across borders (Fraser, 2008; Fraser et al., 2004). It could only be removed by transforming or improving governance structures and decision-making procedures to give people representation through international human rights protocols and by participation (McNay, 2008). Fraser argued that the frame of social justice had expanded beyond nations due to globalisation and international migration (Fraser, 2008). However, this trend was often neglected in programmes to achieve justice and resulted in misframing which, in turn, led to the subordination of the most pressing needs of marginalised groups in society, such as refugees, creating the need for nations to embrace justice frameworks promoted by international organisations, such the UN (Hölscher, 2014). In South Africa, Hölscher (2014) confirmed the central role of Fraser's concept of misframing in her research on social justice and refugees.

Parity of participation: connecting the three axes of social justice

Fraser's theory of social justice maintained that, for social justice to occur, economic (maldistribution), cultural (misrecognition), and political (misrepresentation) factors must all be addressed. Fraser argued that to remedy injustice, marginalised groups had to participate as peers economically, culturally and politically. This brought a core dimension of Fraser's theory that cuts across all three forms of justice and their remedies, all of which were central to the claims of people with disability, namely, parity of participation. It is to this the discussion now turns.

Fraser argued that social justice did not require group recognition but recognition of the status of individuals making up a group or of the group itself relative to other groups (Fraser, 2001). Taken in the context of disability, this meant recognising individuals not only as unique actors who were being denied the opportunity to participate as equals in society, but also groups of people being stigmatised because of their differences. Fraser (2001) argued for 'parity of participation' which allowed 'all (adult) members of society to interact with one another as peers' (p. 6). This meant participation in economic (redistribution), cultural (recognition), and political (representation) forums. Redistribution involved dealing with welfare dependence, inequality, deprivation, exploitation, and other factors that denied people opportunities to interact with their equals as peers (Fraser, 2008, 2010). Parity of participation required acceptance of differences, respect for diverse identities, and equal treatment. Justice required fair interaction in society so all could participate as peers to dismantle 'patterns of advantage and disadvantage that systematically prevent some people from participating on terms of parity' (Fraser et al., 2004, p. 378). Fraser argued that injustice pertained, 'by definition to social institutions and social structures' (Fraser et al., 2004, p. 378) and the barriers that prevented marginalised individuals and groups from participating as peers (Danermark & Coniavitis, 2004).

While participation binds the three axes and makes Fraser's ideas more practical, critics of Fraser's theory of social justice, such as Honneth, have not been happy with her ideas on recognition. As already mentioned, Honneth (1997) initially argued that Fraser's theory did not fully recognise the most important axes of status subordination in society, namely, gender, race, disability, ethnicity and religion. However, these were all later addressed.

Fraser's three axes were intertwined, creating a vicious circle of injustice though, at times, presented competing solutions (Fraser, 2008). For example, recognition called for some groups to be 'recognised' as groups, yet distribution called for the removal of such differentiation. To illustrate, the women's movement called for the abolition of divisions of labour to make men and women equal, as well as recognition of differences between the sexes (Fraser, 2008). Fraser (2008) termed this the redistribution-recognition dilemma, which lay in whether to reinforce or transform societal structures that perpetuated injustice. The call for multicultural societies was an example of the attempt to dilute differences, while indigenisation and decolonisation sought to reclaim cultural heritages lost during colonisation (Fraser, 2008). In spite of these shortcomings, Hölscher (2014) showed that Fraser's theory 'looks set to enrich social work's commitmWent to social justice both in normative and practical terms' (p. 20). As shown in the next section, Fraser's theory provides a rich understanding of misframing and disability injustice.

In the medical fraternity, patients, including those with epilepsy are often treated as subjects, whose role is to receive treatment and care. Ideas about service-user empowerment often lack, especially in the Global South but throughout the world. Medical injustice reinforces power imbalances between healthcare providers and people with epilepsy. For example, in Mozambique, many individuals with epilepsy face significant challenges due to inadequate healthcare infrastructure and limited access to specialised care. They often encounter stigma and discrimination, which can prevent them from receiving appropriate treatment and support. Similarly, in the Middle East, organisations like the Morocco League Against Epilepsy work to address these challenges by promoting awareness, advocating for better healthcare access, and empowering individuals with epilepsy (Kissani et al., 2020). When individuals with epilepsy are not seen as active partners in their care, their needs and perspectives may be overlooked, resulting in impersonal and inadequate treatment. Addressing medical injustice involves recognising people with epilepsy as essential participants in the healthcare process, valuing their input, and incorporating their experiences into treatment planning. This approach aligns with Freire's focus on liberation, Fraser's emphasis on genuine participation, and Ubuntu's view of treating everyone with respect.

Conclusion

This chapter drew on different perspectives to understand the disadvantaging nature of epilepsy—stigma, injustice, disability and death. The stigma perspective argues that society has agreed that epilepsy is an undesirable condition, therefore, people with the condition are less human. This view creates disadvantages for people with epilepsy. The social justice perspectives too see the disadvantage people with epilepsy face as emanating from society. All the perspectives acknowledge the importance of people with epilepsy to be involved in their treatment and care, and for their potential to realised.

References

Amjad, R. N., Nasrabadi, A. N., & Navab, E. (2017). Family stigma associated with epilepsy: A qualitative study. *Journal of Caring Science, 6*(1), 59–65. doi:10.15171/jcs.2017.007

Baskind, R., & Birbeck, G. L. (2005a). Epilepsy care in Zambia: A study of traditional healers. *Epilepsia, 46*(7), 1121–1126. doi:10.1111/j.1528-1167.2005.03505.x

Baskind, R., & Birbeck, G. L. (2005b). Epilepsy-associated stigma in sub-Saharan Africa: The social landscape of a disease. *Epilepsy & Behavior, 7*(1), 68–73. doi:10.1016/j.yebeh.2005.04.009

Birbeck, G. L. (2000). Seizures in rural Zambia. *Epilepsia, 41*(3), 277–281.

Birbeck, G. L., Chomba, E., Atadzhanov, M., Mbewe, E., & Haworth, A. (2006). Zambian teachers: What do they know about epilepsy and how can we work with them to decrease stigma? *Epilepsy & Behavior, 9*(2), 275–280. doi:10.1016/j.yebeh.2006.06.005

Calvert, S. (2011) Epilepsy and disability. National centre for young people with epilepsy. Retrieved May 31, 2017 from https://www.epilepsy.org.au/sites/default/files/Epilepsy%20 and%20Disability%20-%20Sophie%20Calvert.pdf

Caria, S., & Domínguez, R. (2016). Ecuador's "Buen vivir": A new ideology for development. *Latin American Perspectives, 43*(1), 18–33. doi:10.1177/0094582X15611126

Chomba, E. N., Haworth, A., Atadzhanov, M., Mbewe, E., & Birbeck, G. L. (2007). Zambian health care workers' knowledge, attitudes, beliefs, and practices regarding epilepsy. *Epilepsy & Behavior, 10*(1), 111–119.

Danermark, B., & Coniavitis, L. G. (2004). Social justice: Redistribution and recognition-a non-reductionist perspective on disability. *Disability and Society, 19*(4), 339–353.

de Boer, H. M. (2010). Epilepsy stigma: Moving from a global problem to global solutions. *Seizure, 19*(10), 630–636. doi:10.1016/j.seizure.2010.10.017

Dekker, P. A. (2002). *Epilepsy a manual for medical and clinical officers in Africa* (Revised ed.). Geneva: WHO.

Devinsky, O., Vezzani, A., O'Brien, T. J., Jette, N., & Scheffer, I. E. (2018). Epilepsy. The *Lancet, 391*(10122), 342–355.

Dewa, E., January, J., Nyati-Jokomo, Z., Mafaune, P. T., Muteti, S., & Maradzika, J. (2014). Non-attendance of treatment review visits among epileptic patients in a rural district, Zimbabwe. *Journal of Public Health in Africa, 5*(2), 73–76. doi:10.4081/ jphia.2014.351

Duggan, M. B. (2013). Epilepsy and its effects on children and families in rural Uganda. *African Health Sciences, 13*(3), 613–623. doi:10.4314/ahs.v13i3.14

Duvert, C. (2018). How is justice understood in classic Confucianism? *Asian Philosophy, 28*(4), 295–315. doi:10.1080/09552367.2018.1535477

Epilepsy South Africa (ESA). (2014). eDESS (Epilepsy Disability Employment Support Services). Cape town: ESA.

Fraser, N. (1995). From redistribution to recognition? Dilemmas of justice in a 'post-socialist' age. *New Left Review, 212*, 68–93.

Fraser, N. (2000). Rethinking recognition. *New Left Review, 3*(May–June), 107–120.

Fraser, N. (2001). *Social justice in the knowledge society: Redistribution, recognition and participation.* Berlin: Heinrich Boll Stiftung.

Fraser, N. (2003). Social justice in the age of identity politics: Redistribution, recognition and participation. In N. F. A. Honneth (Ed.), *Redistribution or recognition? A political-philosophical exchange* (pp. 7–109). London: Verso.

Fraser, N. (2008). *Scales of justice. Reimaging political space in a globalizing world.* Cambridge: Polity Press.

Fraser, N. (2009). Feminism, capitalisn and the cunning history. *New Left Review, 56*(March–April), 97–117.

Fraser, N. (2010). *Scales of justice: Reimagining political space in a globalising world.* New York: Columbia University Press.

Fraser, N., Dahl, H. M., Stoltz, P., & Willig, R. (2004). Recognition, redistribution and representation in capitalist global society: An interview. *Acta Sociologica, 47*(4), 374–382.

Fraser, N., & Honneth, A. (2003). *Redistribution or recognition? A political-philosophical exchange.* London: Verso.

Freire, P. (1970). *Pedagogy of the oppressed.* Brazil: Herder and Herder.

Freire, P. (1994). *Pedagogy of hope: Reliving pedagogy of the oppressed.* London: Continuum.

Goffman, E. (1963). *Stigma: Notes on the management of a spoiled identity.* New Jersey: Prentice Hall.

Government of South Africa. (1998). *Employment Equity Act*. Cape Town: Government of South Africa.

Government of Zimbabwe. (1992). *Disabled Persons Act*. Harare: Government of Zimbabwe.

Hesdorffer, D. C., Tomson, T., Benn, E. K., & Sander, J. W. (2011). Use of antiepileptic drugs and risk of death: A review. *Epilepsia, 52*(12), 2150–2158. doi:10.1111/j.1528-1167. 2011.03304.x

Hölscher, D. (2014). Considering Nancy Fraser's notion of social justice for Social Work: Reflections on misframing and the lives of refugees in South Africa. *Ethics and Social Welfare, 8*(1), 20–38. doi:10.1080/17496535.2012.744845

Honneth, A. (1997). Recognition and moral obligation. *Social Research, 64*(1), 16–35.

Honneth, A. (2001). Recognition or redistribution? Changing perpectives of the moral order of society. *Theory, Culture & Society, 18*(2–3), 43.

Hunt, P. (1966) *Stigma: The experience of disability*. London: Geoffrey Chapman. Retrieved Novemmber 4, 2016 from https://disability-studies.leeds.ac.uk/library

Kilinc, S., & Campbell, C. (2009). "It shouldn't be something that's evil, it should be talked about": A phenomenological approach to epilepsy and stigma. *Seizure, 18*(10), 665–671. doi:10.1016/j.seizure.2009.09.001

Kissani, N., Balili, K., Mesraoua, B., Abdulla, F., Bashar, G., Al-Baradie, R., Elsahli, R., Ibrahim, E., Al-Asmi, A., Mounir, N., Kishk, N. A., Harharah, A., Abu Aliqa, A., Honein, A., Arabi, M., & Asadi-Pooya, A. A. (2020). Epilepsy and school in the Middle East and North Africa (MENA) region: The current situation, challenges, and solutions. *Epilepsy & Behavior, 112*, 107325–107325. doi:10.1016/j.yebeh.2020.107325

Knight, A. (2015). Democratizing disability: Achieving inclusion (without assimilation) through "Participatory Parity". *Hypatia, 30*(1), 97–114. doi:10.1111/hypa.12120

Kwan, P., & Brodie, M. J. (2000). Early identification of refractory epilepsy. *New England Journal of Medicine, 342*(5), 314–319. doi:10.1056/NEJM200002033420502

Lhatoo, S. D., & Shorvon, S. D. (2008). Sudden death in epilepsy: A review of the literature. *Epilepsia, 49*(7), 1029–1036. doi:10.1111/j.1528-1167.2008.01562.x

Madzokere, C. (1997). Life experiences of people with epilepsy. A study of Highfield high density residential area in Harare, Zimbabwe. *EPICADEC News (Biannual Newsletter of Foundation Epilepsy Care Developing Countries), 10*(97), 19–21.

Mansir, F. (2022). The study of social justice in Pancasila, Islam, and Hinduism perspective. *Jurnal Ilmiah Pendidikan Pancasila Dan Kewarganegaraan, 7*(2), 342–348. doi:10.17977/um019v7i2p342-348

McNay, L. (2008). The trouble with recognition: Subjectivity, suffering, and agency. *Sociological Theory, 26*(3), 271–296. doi:10.1111/j.1467-9558.2008.00329.x

Meinardi, H., Scott, R. A., Reis, R., & Sander, J. W. (2001). The treatment gap in epilepsy: The current situation and ways forward. *Epilepsia, 42*(1), 136–149.

Mladenov, T. (2016). Disability and social justice. *Disability & Society, 31*(9), 1226–1241. doi:10.1080/09687599.2016.1256273

Morrison, Z. (2010). *On dignity: Social inclusion and the politics of recognition* (Volume 1 Social Policy Working Paper). Melbourne: Brotherhood of St Laurence and Centre for Public Policy.

Mtetwa, E. (2011). Policy dimensions of exclusion: Disability as charity and not right in Zimbabwe. *Indian Journal of Social Work, 72*(3), 381–398.

Mugumbate, J., & Nyanguru, A., (2013). Exploring African philosophy: The value of Ubuntu in Social Work. *African Journal of Social Work, 3*(1), 82–100.

Murove, M. F. (2007). The Shona ethic of Ukama with reference to the immortality of values. *Mankind Quarterly, 48*(2), 179–189.

Mushi, D., Hunter, E., Mtuya, C., Mshana, G., Aris, E. & Walker, R. (2011). Social-cultural aspects of epilepsy in Kilimanjaro Region, Tanzania: Knowledge and experience among patients and carers. *Epilepsy and Behaviour, 20*, 338–343.

Ndoye, N. F., Sow, A. D., Diop, A. G., Sessouma, B., Séne-Diouf, F., Boissy, L.,..., & Sander, J. W. A. S. (2005). Prevalence of epilepsy its treatment gap and knowledge, attitude and practice of its population in sub-urban Senegal an ILAE/IBE/WHO study. *Seizure: European Journal of Epilepsy, 14*, 106–111. doi:10.1016/j.seizure.2004.11.003

Newton, C. R., & Garcia, H. H. (2012). Epilepsy in poor regions of the world. *Lancet, 380*(9848), 1193–1201. doi:10.1016/s0140-6736(12)61381-6

Nuhu, F. T., Fawole, J. O., Babalola, O. J., Ayilara, O. O., & Sulaiman, Z. T. (2010). Social consequences of epilepsy: A study of 231 Nigerian patients. *Annals of African Medicine, 9*(3), 170–175. doi:10.4103/1596-3519.68360

Obeid, T. (2008). Stigma: An aspect of epilepsy not to be ignored. *Saudi Medical Journal, 29*(4), 489–497.

Ochs, P. (2012). Competing for Abrahamic Justice. *Religions (Dawḥah, Qatar), 2012*(2). doi:10.5339/rels.2012.justice.12

Oliver, M. (2013). *The social model of disablility: Thirty years on* (Vol. 28). Oxfordshire: Carfax International.

Reis, R., & Meinardi, H. (2002). ILAE/WHO "Out of the Shadows Campaign" Stigma: Does the flag identify the cargo? *Epilepsy & Behavior, 3*, 33.

Samkange, S. J. W. T., & Samkange, S. (1980). *Hunhuism or Ubuntuism: A Zimbabwe indigenous political philosophy*. Harare: Graham.

Scambler, G. (2009) Health-related stigma. *Sociology of Health & Illness, 31*(3), 441–455.

Sen, A. (1985a). *Commodities and capabilities*. Amsterdam: Elsevier.

Sen, A. (1985b). *Well-being, agency, and freedom: Poverty and inequality*. Oxford: Oxford University Press.

Shava, K. (2008). *How and in what ways can Western models of disability inform and promote the empowerment of disabled people and their participation in mainstream Zimbabwean society?* (Degree of Masters of Arts in Disability Studies). Leeds: University of Leeds.

Taylor, C. (1994). The politics of recognition. In A. Gutman (Ed.), *Multiculturalism* (pp. 25–74). Princeton, NJ: Princeton University Press.

Tellez-Zenteno, J. F., & Hernandez-Ronquillo, L. (2012). Mortality in epilepsy. *Current Neurology and Neuroscience Reports, 12*(3), 345–351.

United Nations (UN). (2000). *Millennium declaration*. New York: UN.

United Nations (UN). (2006). *Convention on the rights of persons with disabilities*. New York: UN.

Venugopal, C. N. (2013). Polity, religion and secularism in India: A study of interrelationships. *Politikologija Religije, 7*(1), 21–40. doi:10.54561/prj0701021v

Vos, T., Faxman, A. D., & Naghavi, M. (2012). Years lived with disability (YLDs) for 1160 sequelae of 289 diseases and injuries 1990–2010: A systematic analysis for the Global Burden of Disease Study 2010. *Lancet, 380*, 2163–2196

Wasserman, D., Asch, A., Blustein, J., & Putnam, D. (2015). Disability and justice. In E. N. Zalta (Ed.), *The stanford encyclopedia of philosophy* (Summer ed.). Retrieved July 16, 2017 from https://plato.stanford.edu/archives/sum2015/entries/disability-justice/

Watts, A. E. (1989). A model for managing epilepsy in a rural community in Africa. *British Medical Journal, 298*, 235–268. doi:10.1136/bmj.298.6676.805

Watts, A. E. (1992). The natural history of untreated epilepsy in a rural community in Africa. *Epilepsia, 33*(3), 464–468.

Wilmshurst, J. M., Kakooza-Mwesige, A., & Newton, C. R. (2014). The challenges of managing children with epilepsy in Africa. *Seminars in Pediatric Neurology, 21*, 36–41. doi:10.1016/j.spen.2014.01.005

World Health Organisation (WHO). (2011). *World report on disability*. Retrieved August 13, 2014 from https://www.who.int/disabilities/world_report/2011/en/

World Health Organisation (WHO). (2016). *Epilepsy*. Retrieved October 16, 2016. from https://www.who.int/mediacentre/factsheets/fs999/en/

6 Multiple impacts and responses in resource-poor settings

The disadvantages of epilepsy present multiple direct impacts on people with the condition. This chapter discusses these multiple impacts of living with in resource-poor settings and responses with examples from a study that was completed in Zimbabwe, Africa. The qualitative study used in-depth interviews with 16 unemployed and 14 employed people with epilepsy (n = 30), who were members of the Epilepsy Support Foundation (ESF) in Harare, Zimbabwe's capital. Participants comprised of 13 females and 17 males with a mean age of 33 years. To deepen understanding of the interview findings, the perspectives of ESF service providers (n = 7) were sought through a focus group discussion. The service providers included two health workers, three social service workers and two advocacy workers. The two datasets were analysed separately using NVivo, a computer-assisted, qualitative data-analysis package. As in many other countries in the Global South, where public services are less than ideal, people with epilepsy in Zimbabwe encounter difficulties in obtaining social support and employment assistance. This chapter focuses on impacts of negative beliefs about epilepsy, gaps in public services, job-seeking and workplace environment, self-management and individual factors will be discussed. This chapter ends with a discussion of the study's implications for social policy, epilepsy work and social work (Table 6.1).

Summary of findings from the study

Table 6.1 Key findings from the Zimbabwe study

Findings	Details
Negative impact of beliefs about epilepsy	Dominant understandings of epilepsy led to social exclusion.
	Persistent trust in ineffective healing—led to delayed seizure control.
Ongoing gaps in public services	Lack of educational and vocational support services.
	Lack of public social welfare and public disability services.
	Medical health services were expensive and difficult to access.
	Reliance on non-government support services.

(Continued)

DOI: 10.4324/9781003602866-6

Table 6.1 (Continued)

Findings	Details
Challenging job-seeking and workplace environment	Job-seeking challenges.
	Persistent barriers in the workplace.
	Gender issues in the workplace.
	Absence of employment services.
	Lack of recourse to justice in the workplace.
Self-management and individual factors	Self-management, resilience and vulnerability.
	Individual factors.
Effective strategies	Epilepsy education.
	Government services.
	Non-government services.

Negative impact of beliefs about epilepsy

Misunderstanding, inaccurate cultural and religious beliefs persisted that epilepsy was caused by, and manifested, an evil or avenging supernatural spirit. People with epilepsy, seen as mediums of evil spirits were, therefore, feared. These inaccurate beliefs had detrimental effects and contributed to a devaluing of people with epilepsy in their families, community, school and workplace. Family members, friends, neighbours, teachers, health workers, employers, co-workers and the general community harboured negative views of epilepsy. Hence, epileptic seizures became a mark of undesirability in society, resulting in social stigma.

In Zimbabwe, stigma was institutionalised in Christian churches and Indigenous cultures. It served no other purpose than being a conduit of social exclusion. People with epilepsy and service providers who participated in the study agreed that a sequence of barriers culminated in poor employment outcomes for people with epilepsy. At the base of this sequence lay cultural and religious beliefs that sustained ineffective traditional treatment practices for epilepsy. These beliefs fostered negative social attitudes that resulted in fear, stigma, and exclusion, leading to delayed medical treatment, and compromised education and vocational training— key factors for positive employment outcomes. This was compounded by poor public services. Hence, the chances of attaining or maintaining employment were reduced.

The Zimbabwe study confirmed prior findings on the role of negative social attitudes in reducing the quality of life of people with epilepsy in Zimbabwe (Madzokere, 1997; Mielke, Adamolekun, Ball, & Mundanda, 1997; Mugumbate & Mushonga, 2013; Saburi, Mapanga, & Mapanga, 2006), in other African countries (Birbeck, 2000; Duggan, 2013; Halima et al., 2017; Hounsossou et al., 2015; Keikelame & Swartz, 2015; Mushi et al., 2011; Nuhu, Fawole, Babalola, Ayilara, & Sulaiman, 2010; Watts, 1989, 1992) and worldwide (Baskind & Birbeck, 2005a; Bishop, 2002; Elger & Schmidt, 2008; Kilinc & Campbell, 2009; Meinardi, Scott, Reis, & Sander, 2001; WHO, 2015). In Senegal, Halima et al. (2017) found that employed people with epilepsy were feared and looked down upon and this impacted on finding work and job promotion. Findings related to these were found in Benin, where Hounsossou et al. (2015) reported that epilepsy was considered contagious, which reduced willingness to employ people with epilepsy. In Malaysia, Wo, Lim, Choo and Tan (2016) found that stigma lowered employment. In this study, negative social attitudes were found to act as barriers to socialisation, treatment, education, training and employment opportunities for people with epilepsy. For most, persistent ignorance about epilepsy had led to stigmatisation and isolation and ongoing fears, not only in the workplace, but also in school. Headmasters, teachers and fellow pupils feared people with epilepsy, which led to their social exclusion. Bishop (2002) reported similar findings found in Senegal and Malaysia. In Zimbabwe, as in all these countries, persistent misunderstanding of epilepsy was a major barrier to employment.

In the Zimbabwe study, service providers were all too aware of these barriers to social inclusion for people with epilepsy, highlighting International Labour Organisation's (ILO) (2015) view that community-based, non-government services, such as those provided by ESF, were extremely important for people with epilepsy. ESF played an important role in educating people with epilepsy and their families, giving them access to treatment and support. Awareness enhanced understanding of epilepsy as a medical condition and increased treatment uptake and control of seizures to counter the social exclusion and isolation of people with epilepsy. However, many people in Zimbabwe harboured negative social attitudes bolstered by unscientific and superstitious religious and cultural beliefs. It was, therefore, unsurprising that people continued to fear epilepsy and its consequences. These beliefs formed the basis for cultural and religious interventions, resulting in the seemingly endless competition between traditional and medical treatment.

Persistent trust in ineffective healing led to delayed seizure control

Traditional treatment, which included cultural and religious interventions, was the first port of call in line with local beliefs. This confirms previous findings in Zimbabwe (Adamolekun, Mielke, & Ball, 1999; Mutanana & Mutara, 2015). This situation was not peculiar to Zimbabwe, but existed in African countries like Nigeria, Uganda, Tanzania, Zambia and Malawi (Birbeck, 2000; Duggan, 2013; Mushi et al., 2011; Nuhu et al., 2010; Watts, 1989, 1992). ILO (2015, 2017) argued that negative attitudes towards people with disability result in poor employment outcomes. There were several reasons for this trend in this study. First, the reliance on cultural remedies and religious solutions was as much a factor of some erroneous beliefs as of their ready availability within the community, as well as the tremendous power enjoyed by traditional healers in Zimbabwe. Second, cultural and religious healing was a well-embedded social institution and an industry that generated livelihoods for its practitioners – prophets, church owners, traditional healers and herbalists, who were legitimate authorities (Chitando, Gunda, & Kügler, 2013; Watts, 1989). Third, for people with epilepsy and their families, these cultural and religious healing practices offered an accessible, affordable solution, made more attractive by the lack of affordable medical treatment (Magazi, 2017). Ready access to traditional treatment led to delayed medical treatment, which, in turn, led not only to social problems relating to education, training and employment, but also to psychological and mental health issues and social isolation (de Boer, 2010; Elger & Schmidt, 2008; International League Against Epilepsy [ILAE], World Health Organisation [WHO], & International Bureau for Epilepsy [IBE], 2000; Meinardi et al., 2001). Fourth, through attending traditional ceremonies and events such as church gatherings, psychosocial support was provided to people with epilepsy, and this was important given the lack of psychosocial support initiatives such as counselling. This explanation would fit participants prior to visiting the ESF. Fifth, but not least, traditional healers offered hope and usually promised quick healing, including apportioning blame to witches (Chitando et al., 2013; Jackson & Mupedziswa, 1988).

The focus group discussion provided new insights into why people with epilepsy delayed medical treatment in favour of traditional treatments: taking medicines, especially for prolonged periods, was not favourable, and was often discouraged in Zimbabwean society. Because of this, medical treatment was taken at the last resort. And even so, medical treatment was often stopped. This sounds like a plausible explanation for delays in getting medical treatment and reasons for defaulting medical treatment. However, there could still be other reasons making this possible. These include poor public services. The lack of public services represented economic injustice, especially so considering that HIV and AIDS programmes and other politically expedient programmes were being adequately funded by the government.

There was competition between traditional and medical treatments in Zimbabwe, as in Africa generally (Magazi, 2017; WHO, 2016; Winkler et al., 2009). This competition rested on several factors. First, people with epilepsy continued to use traditional treatments, which service providers did not promote and health workers did not overtly though might clandestinely support them due to their cultural embeddedness. Secondly, Zimbabwe's laws and institutions promoted the use of traditional and medical treatments. People with epilepsy, and Zimbabweans in general, were caught between two worlds: the scientific, where medical treatment has proven effectiveness in controlling epilepsy and sociocultural, where traditional and religious practices encourage ineffective treatments undergirded by strongly held beliefs in the supernatural. Thirdly, traditional treatment practice has proved remarkably resilient in the face of strong competition for market share from medical practice and pharmacological industries. Both are profitable economic ventures, competing for the business of people with epilepsy. The other type of competition was between Indigenous and Christian treatments themselves. However, since this competition reduced opportunities for achieving a better quality of life for people with epilepsy, complementarity, rather than competition, is desirable.

Traditional treatments were ineffective, and in other cases costly but they were pursued nonetheless. The reasons given by participants for reliance on traditional treatments point to the strength of beliefs and the shortcomings of medical treatment (Jackson & Mupedziswa, 1988; Mutanana & Mutara, 2015). First, despite the shortcomings of traditional treatments, their social value and the power of traditional healers were still strong, one reason why medical interventions failed to change beliefs in traditional treatments (Jackson & Mupedziswa, 1988). The presence of evil spirits was well embedded in the Zimbabwean psyche (Dube, Shoko, & Haves, 2011; Jackson & Mupedziswa, 1988; Madzokere, 1997; Mutanana & Mutara, 2015). Thus, identifying witches, who were purveyors of evil spirits, allowed the family to accord blame and find an outlet for their anger and possibly reduce stigma in the process. This could as well have reduced stigma attached to the family. Further, the survival of *Chivanhu* depended on people's persistent belief in the supernatural. Second, in the absence of psychosocial support services such as counselling and group work, religious and cultural gatherings closed the gap. Third, the lack of affordable and readily accessible medical treatment services meant traditional treatments were better option. However, the inefficacy of traditional treatments led to persistent seizures.

In the Zimbabwe study, with appropriate medical treatment, seizure control facilitated improved educational, training, and job opportunities and greater acceptance in the workplace and wider community. Many of the participants had first learnt about medical treatment from the ESF in Harare, but most people with epilepsy in Zimbabwe were severely disadvantaged by the prevalence of ignorance about epilepsy and the absence of appropriate medical resources, especially in rural areas (Madzokere, 1997; Mutanana & Mutara, 2015). On face value, it sounds like medical treatment was all what was needed to improve opportunities but the journey from the first seizure to getting medical treatment was very long due to beliefs and the absence of easily accessible and affordable treatment services as already discussed.

Use of traditional treatment resulted from a lack of affordable, accessible, quality healthcare and, most importantly, community education and awareness of epilepsy as an easily treatable neurological condition (Baskind & Birbeck, 2005a; ILAE et al., 2000; Meinardi et al., 2001). In some instances, participants reported that health service providers like nurses, who well knew that epilepsy was a treatable condition, encouraged people to seek traditional treatments. On a broader level, failure to control seizures is related to gaps in public services. Not only were policies inadequate, but services were poor and this impacted negatively on educational and employment opportunities for people with epilepsy.

Ongoing gaps in public services

Lack of educational and vocational support services

Consistent with the literature, people with epilepsy reported lack of educational and vocational qualifications (Abidi & Sharma, 2014; Banks & Polack, 2015; Échevin, 2013; Halima et al., 2017; Liao & Zhao, 2013; Schur, Kruse, Blasi, & Blanck, 2009; Wolffe, Ajuwon, & Kelly, 2013). Due to misinformation and stigma, the participants experienced barriers to education. Consequently, participants with childhood-onset epilepsy reported limited access to primary and secondary school education. Some had attended sporadically, while others had been forced to drop out of school. Some teachers did not know about medical treatment or did not support it, and encouraged their students with epilepsy to seek favoured traditional interventions. Services to support vocational training were equally lacking. None of the participants had benefited from the government-run vocational training schemes, apprenticeships, cadetships, scholarships and human-resource development. Service providers were critical of government rehabilitation services, such as Ruwa Rehabilitation Centre, near Harare, which offered medical rehabilitation and job-skills training. Its capacity was low, it was highly selective, and favoured people with physical disabilities.

It was clear from the experiences of participants in the Zimbabwe study that educational institutions did not have academic inclusion plans to meet the needs of people with epilepsy which should be standard practice in modern institutions of learning. Without these plans, people with disability fail to learn productively, at times they fail courses and this delays their completion. At the end, they fail not because they are not intelligent, but because enough attention is not given to the disadvantage they already have. Without plans to ensure inclusion, people with epilepsy were excluded from participation and did not enter the labour market.

Lack of public social welfare and disability services

In the Zimbabwe study, not only were welfare and disability services not available, but also accessing public services presented difficulties because the families of most participants were poor. Without extra assistance from the government, they could not meet their basic needs for health, education and food, let alone gain employment skills or startup capital for informal enterprises. None of the participants was receiving social assistance from the government even though the Social Welfare Assistance Act (Government of Zimbabwe, 1988) and the Disabled Persons Act (Government of Zimbabwe, 1992) provided for monthly means-tested disability grants of US$20. Since these depended on the type and severity of the disability, people with epilepsy were often excluded, as they did not have recognisable impairments. People with physical disabilities, such as those without sight and limbs, were more likely to be eligible for disability grants than those with hidden neurological and cognitive disabilities. Grants were a form of social security that helped reduce poverty and address the challenges that prevented people with disabilities from participating in the labour market (Banks & Polack, 2015; Buckup, 2002; ILO, 2006; Mtetwa, 2011). However, it has been argued that, while welfare grants alleviated poverty in South Africa, they reduced employment-seeking behaviour and therefore failed to provide a long-term solution (Sung, Muller, Jones, & Fong, 2014; Schneider, Mokomane, & Graham, 2016). Service providers in this study confirmed that, without disability support, people with epilepsy found it difficult to provide for their basic health and education needs and, in most instances, their families could not provide for their skills training.

The service providers reported that the disability grant was supposed to be disbursed to district social welfare offices by the treasury on monthly or annually but most districts had not received funds for several years, confirming what previous researched termed a lack of political will in Zimbabwe (Choruma, 2006; Lang & Charowa, 2007; Marongwe & Mate, 2007; SINTEF, 2003). The country's economic difficulties notwithstanding, welfare clients in receipt of other welfare grants were receiving regular payments. War veterans were a case in point. They included those who had fought in the war of liberation that had ended with Zimbabwe's independence in 1980. They were receiving US$360 monthly for welfare support, 18 times more than recipients of disability grants. Clearly, there were strong political factors at work here, since this constituted the ruling government's power base. Seen through Fraser's lens of social justice, people with epilepsy lacked recognition and representation, that is, social and political power respectively. Not only was the disability payment abysmally low at US$20 monthly, but the means test excluded most people with epilepsy. To promote employment creation for disadvantaged groups, the Zimbabwean government distributed US$500 annually to districts for developmental projects, such as small enterprise development. This could do little given most districts comprised about 200,000 people and monies for individual and group support was rarely made available or would be diverted to other uses or simply misused by government officials.

From the Zimbabwe study, it was clear that the government was not resourcing local or nationwide awareness initiatives and was not prioritising disability in the allocation of national resources, as shown by the non-availability of public social assistance for participants in this study. Instead, the government prioritised the politically expedient war veterans' pension. This constituted a maldistribution of public resources, which was rampant in Zimbabwe, fuelled by corruption and the mismanagement of public resources (Transparency International Zimbabwe, 2015).

Service providers and participants agreed that epilepsy was neglected both as a disability and chronic health condition. They recommended that the Disabled Persons Act (Government of Zimbabwe, 1992) should recognise epilepsy as a disability to ensure the inclusion of people with epilepsy in government programmes. However, not all people with epilepsy experienced disabilities, especially where epilepsy was treated and reasonable accommodations achieved. To that end, it was important that disability legislation recognised all impairments, including epilepsy, based on a clear definition of the type of limitations that constitute a disability.

Disability services lacked a central case-management system so welfare services were divorced from employment support, yet success hinged on collaboration between service providers. The National Disability Board, which ran the National Disability Fund, had no dedicated staff and depended on Department of Social Welfare officials, who were overwhelmed with other duties. Literature persistently showed that employment support was an important pillar that promoted successful employment outcomes for people with epilepsy (Buckup, 2009; ILO, 2016; Soeker, Van Rensburg, & Travill, 2012; Yuh, Yun-Tung, Meng-Hsiu, & Shih, 2013).

Medical health services were expensive and difficult to access

Results from the Zimbabwe study showed that health services were of poor quality and expensive, and therefore, beyond reach for most participants in this study.

Consistent with findings from two studies in Malawi and many other African countries, people with epilepsy in Zimbabwe delayed treatment by several years (Baskind & Birbeck, 2005a; Elger & Schmidt, 2008; Mushi et al., 2011; Watts, 1989, 1992; WHO, 2016). Medicines and vital medical services were often not available and, when they were, were expensive. Though public health services were available in urban areas, their quality was erratic. Hospitals were overcrowded and under-resourced and the community health workforce lacked the capacity to complement hospital-based treatment or to educate communities about epilepsy and the ease with which it could be treated, if properly understood as a neurological condition. Another factor that compromised health services related to health personnel, notably the fact that there was no neurologist available in Zimbabwe at the time of the research. Service providers pointed out that nurses were not appropriately trained to manage epilepsy yet patients were attended to by nurses most of the time. Many a time, nurses waited for doctors to diagnose and initiate treatment for epilepsy, increasing the time patients had to wait before they got initial medical treatment. Issues of poor health services and inadequately trained nurses have been reported in previous studies in Zimbabwe and other African countries (Baskind & Birbeck, 2005a; Duggan, 2013; Mushi et al., 2011; Saburi et al., 2006).

Reliance on non-government support services

As already mentioned, all participants had received non-government services, including counselling, treatment, information, training and (limited) employment support services from the ESF. Service providers at the ESF indicated that resource-strapped NGOs had assumed several roles usually filled by government services. They highlighted that, given more nurses, social workers and community workers, the ESF could provide treatment for more people with epilepsy and improve the quality of life of those already on treatment. However, the consensus was that the organisation was too small to cover the whole nation. Hence, the provision of public services to people with epilepsy remained a public-sector duty that government should prioritise. It was clear from the focus group discussion that service providers did not have the requisite skills to provide effective, planned, long-term employment services. Literature shows that that non-government organisations played an important role in improving the quality of life of people with epilepsy, together with reliable public services (2015; Jacoby & Baker, 2008; WHO, 2016).

Challenging job-seeking and workplace environment

Job-seeking challenges

Three main factors made job-seeking challenging—lack of vocational skills, uncontrolled seizures and competition for limited job opportunities. With seizures, job seekers with epilepsy could not easily hide their condition. Once noticed and labelled, they would not easily find employment. Their job networks dwindled and having qualifications carried little weight once it was known they had epilepsy. However, some with controlled seizures lacked appropriate vocational training, and did not have the requisite work skills required by employers. This made it very difficult for them to succeed in a highly competitive job market. When jobs were available, these were undesirable and characterised by low pay.

As in many countries in the Global South, there was a lack of employment opportunities and no employment quota system for people with disability, just like in Zimbabwe. Literature shows that reserving positions for people with disabilities reduced barriers to employment (Abidi & Sharma, 2014; Échevin, 2013; Schur et al., 2009). The Zimbabwean government's policy on equalisation of opportunities for people with disability in the public sector only supported those already in public employment and did not cover those in private employment (Government of Zimbabwe, 2011). South Africa offered an example: its government had reserved 2% of jobs in the public service for people with disabilities (Gathiram, 2008). This figure, though low, given that 15% of employees were expected to have disabilities, was at least a starting point.

There was no doubt Zimbabwe's economic decline that had seen many companies closing, scaling back, or migrating to other countries, could account for the lack of job opportunities but this did not explain the exclusion of people with epilepsy from the same market that accommodated their peers and siblings. Official government statistics reported an unemployment rate of 11%, when the majority of the economically active population was 'employed' in the informal agriculture and trade (Government of Zimbabwe, 2012). For people with epilepsy, penetrating this informal job market was equally difficult, due to negative attitudes and lack of skills or capital to start informal businesses. For those with formal jobs, persistent barriers made their employment situation tenuous; many were in jobs where their skills were underused meaning they were unproductively employed.

Persistent barriers in the workplace

Not only had participants faced barriers to treatment and education, due to negative social attitudes but also in the workplace, where persistent misinformation about epilepsy generated fear and affected their relations with co-workers, managers and customers, as the case might be. In the workplace, people believed epilepsy was contagious. There were persistent beliefs that employees with epilepsy were incompetent; employees would leave if they knew a co-worker had epilepsy; customers would be lost; or, at the extreme, the person with epilepsy would die on the job. These persistent beliefs, negative attitudes and resultant fears made it difficult for people with epilepsy to maintain their employment; curtailed their productivity; affected them psychologically resulting in mental health issues and, in some cases, seizures; compromised their earning potential and promotional prospects; led to unfair dismissals; and prevented access to pension and medical aid despite the tenuousness of their employment and retention issues. This confirmed earlier findings pointing to the reluctance of employers to hire people with disability (Buckup, 2002; Halima et al., 2017; Hlatywayo, Hlatywayo, & Mtezo, 2014; Hounsossou et al., 2015; Wiggett-Barnard & Swartz, 2012). This reluctance persisted, despite studies showing the benefits of, and dispelling negative stereotypes about, employing people with epilepsy (Banks & Polack, 2015; Bishop, 2002; Buckup, 2009; ILO, 2016; Jacoby & Baker, 2008; Jacoby, Gorry, & Baker, 2005; van Niekerk, 2010; Wolffe et al., 2013a). However, on a positive note, past experiences of working with people with epilepsy had enhanced employers' willingness to hire and retain them in the same manner reported by Jacoby et al. (2005).

Workplace policies and employer networks to create a receptive environment for hiring and retention were non-existent in Zimbabwean workplaces, yet these were found to be facilitators of employment in an earlier study by Erickson, von Schrader, Bruyère, and VanLooy (2014) and Jacoby et al. (2005). This showed that the presence of labour laws, such as the Labour Act (Government of Zimbabwe, 2005), did not guarantee non-discrimination and fair labour practices. The law was useful only where employers believed people with epilepsy were equal to other employees and that they could work productively. Some employers did not seem to think that it was unfair to dismiss people with epilepsy from work. The same could be said of labour unions, yet they should recognise and protect those facing discrimination, including working women. Employers did not consider this burden, making the needs of women with epilepsy misrecognised.

Gender issues in the workplace

Women reported more burdensome experiences in employment, but there were no discernible gender differences in other experiences like education and job-seeking. Working women with epilepsy reported a 'triple burden' as income earners, mothers and wives, and people living with a disabling chronic condition. This burden increased their risk of dismissal at work, as Mucha's case study clearly demonstrated. Further, in traditional Zimbabwean society, women were expected to take on caring roles in the family and to enter caring professions, such as teaching or nursing (Chifamba, 2015; Peta, McKenzie & Kathard, 2015). This had changed little with the shift to women playing a more active role in the labour market. Despite calls for national and workplace policies that recognised the roles of women and addressed the disadvantages they might face in securing and maintaining employment (Buckup, 2009; ILO, 2016), women in Zimbabwe still faced more barriers than men in the labour market (Chifamba, 2015; Choruma, 2006; Madzokere, 1997; Peta et al., 2015). The situation might become unbearable for them, especially considering the absence of employment support services reported in this study. Women with disability were also disadvantaged in other countries (Banks & Polack, 2015; Buckup, 2002). Fraser and other social justice theorists viewed this as misrecognition that prevented women to participate as peers (Danermark & Coniavitis, 2004; Knight, 2015; McNay, 2008).

Absence of employment services

The social interventions to support employment described in the literature, including occupational services (ILO, 2001, 2015; Soeker et al., 2012), were not available for most participants in this study, neither were there any dedicated government disability employment service. Reports from the department showed that it was severely understaffed, employment officers were overwhelmed with work, and there were no disability-specific services. The ESF and other non-government organisations did not have specific employment services. Studies have shown that economic problems were among the most reported challenges of people with epilepsy (Mugumbate & Nyanguru, 2013) and other disabilities (Cramm, Nieboer, Finkenflügel, & Lorenzo, 2013; Cramm, Lorenzo, & Nieboer, 2014), yet income support services too were lacking for the participants of this study. Previous studies showed that services to support employment reduced barriers for people with disabilities (Banks & Polack, 2015; ILO, 2005; Yuh et al., 2013).

Service providers were not aware of targeted disability schemes run by the Public Service Commission, which recruited government personnel. However, the Commission had a policy to equalise opportunities in the public service which was supposed to be overseen by disability-focused persons in various government departments. The policy ostensibly sought to reduce discrimination for those already in employment and, to a lesser extent, those seeking employment but it had no specific objectives to improve the work skills of jobless people with disabilities. Affirmative action policies might increase access to the recruitment of people with epilepsy but government first needed to ensure the basic human right to education, work and earning a liveable wage was entrenched in its policies and services. Earlier studies found that affirmative action facilitated employment (Banks & Polack, 2015; Maja, Mann, Sing, Steyn, & Naidoo, 2011; Marumoagae, 2012; Mizunoya & Mitra, 2013).

Lack of recourse to justice in the workplace

Despite human rights and labour laws to reduce discrimination and provide policy measures to increase the inclusion of people with disability in the labour market, people with epilepsy remained excluded. In this study, participants were unable to challenge their dismissals or other experiences of discrimination in court. Existing legal channels, such as they were, were expensive with limited chances of success due to the policy environment and negative social attitudes toward people with epilepsy. Effectively, therefore, they had no recourse to justice following unfair dismissals related to seizures in the workplace. For example, while the Labour Court of Zimbabwe was a sound institution, it was not useful because people with epilepsy required huge sums of money to hire lawyers to help them navigate the complex legal system. If they did not hire lawyers, the employers they were challenging would do so, making their legal efforts futile. It took a long time before cases were heard and before judgements were delivered although the Disabled Persons Act (Government of Zimbabwe, 1992) had antidiscrimination clauses, no case had been brought to court indicating that those facing discrimination suffered in silence, as did the participants in this study.

The years wasted on trying to access education, appropriate medical treatment and employment would be the subject of lawsuits in the Global North but, in Zimbabwe, people's expectations of the government had reached an all-time low, due to years of misrecognition of people with disabilities (Honneth, 1997). Not only did the treatment of people with epilepsy in the workplace constitute a violation of their basic human right to work and earn an income, but the lack of recognition and representation for people with disabilities in Zimbabwean society meant an absence of advocacy. Without a strong, collective service-user voice, social injustices persisted (Danermark & Coniavitis, 2004; Fraser, 2001). Without strong advocacy for human rights and social justice, the government was unlikely to reorganise labour and develop effective labour market policies accommodating diverse groups in Zimbabwean society. More particularly, it was unlikely to ensure mechanisms were in place to ensure recourse to justice in the face of unfair work practices and wrongful dismissal. The dire economic situation in Zimbabwe did little to improve educational, health, employment, welfare and legal services. Public service failures resulted in people with epilepsy resorting to self-management to overcome barriers to employment.

Self-management and individual factors

This study found an individualistic service ethos, where individuals had to solve their own problems and where problems were treated on a case-by-case basis. Due to the failure of public support systems and the individualistic service ethos, participants had become self-reliant and resilient; however, some became vulnerable. This argument has been raised before by other researchers (Dewa et al., 2014; Bradley, Lindsay, & Fleeman, 2016; Munn, 2008; Richardson, 2002; Sebit & Mielke, 2005). Several individual factors made this possible.

Self-management, resilience and vulnerability

The findings of this study pointed to a sequence of barriers culminating in poor employment outcomes for people with epilepsy, including fear, stigma and exclusion. This was compounded by poor public services. Hence the chances of attaining or maintaining employment were reduced. In the words of Service Provider 5, success was 'by force or by God's grace'. This resulted in people with epilepsy having to deal with their seizures and socioeconomic injustices. With no reliable public services, people with epilepsy were left to manage their adversity themselves. Some were resilient and succeeded but others became more vulnerable, as had been reported in prior studies (Dewa et al., 2014; Jacoby & Baker, 2008; Munn, 2008; Richardson, 2002; Sebit & Mielke, 2005). Some participants adopted a fighting spirit, while others simply gave up.

Resilient individuals accepted their condition and maintained a positive attitude and had a mastery of epilepsy. They had supportive families and employers. This confirmed prior studies on the importance of support systems in building resilience (Elliott & Shneker, 2008; Ring, Jacob, Baker, Marson, & Whitehead, 2016). Elliott and Shneker (2008) found that health workers who formed part of these support systems lacked correct knowledge about epilepsy. The participants of this study were positive about the ESF and the service providers believed in the importance of support groups, public education and advocacy work. In other rare cases, participants such as Munya reported that their employers were supportive, although co-workers were not. Previous research by Jacoby et al. (2005) concluded that some employers were willing to accommodate people with epilepsy. Factors that promoted this positive attitude were having employed people with epilepsy previously, correct knowledge of epilepsy and having disability support services.

Vulnerability was exacerbated by continuous negative attitudes towards people with epilepsy. Without supportive policies and programmes, vulnerable participants failed to overcome the vast socioeconomic challenges they faced or to secure timely medical treatment. Though interventions focused on individuals, prior studies confirmed that individual vulnerability was related to external factors, such as access to essential resources and services and economic opportunities (Ring et al., 2016). Participants in this study, such as Munya, Hadeel and Derry, had resorted to informal employment, even though it was not rewarding and they lacked the finances to engage fully in productive informal work. Others sought work in neighbouring countries following their failure to secure work in the formal labour market. Their persistence attested their resilience

A mastery of epilepsy and good seizure control were found to be good facilitators of employment in this study confirming previous findings (Al-Adawi et al., 2003; Coker, Bhargava, Fitzgerald, & Doherty, 2011; Elliott & Shneker, 2008; Ring et al., 2016). In this study, seizure control depended on family beliefs, knowledge of epilepsy and treatment accessibility. Unreliable health services led to restricted employment chances for people with epilepsy, as found in other studies (Sebit & Mielke, 2005). This study showed that employment challenges for people with epilepsy were multifaceted and required diverse interventions and supports. In the absence of such supports, individual resilience and self-management became pivotal to coping but were unlikely to offer a total solution for the massive socio-structural, cultural and economic problems impacting on the lives of people with epilepsy in Zimbabwe. Clearly, individual resilience and self-management were coping mechanism but were unlikely to offer a total solution to the problems of people with epilepsy in Zimbabwe. People could cope with social support, but the most important factor in living a quality life was the independence that came with gainful employment.

Individual factors

While the study focused on structural factors impacting employment of people with epilepsy, the experiences showed individual attributes had an influence too. Literature showed that these included mastery of epilepsy, age; seizure onset, type and control; marital status; geographical location; economic status; well-being; and intelligence (Al-Adawi et al., 2003; Coker et al., 2011; Elliott & Shneker, 2008; Tai, 2011; Wo et al., 2016). Some of these were applicable to participants in this study, as already discussed but they are highlighted again here.

Since most participants (n = 18) had child-onset epilepsy, their parents had arranged their treatment, which increased the likelihood of traditional treatment as the first port of call, due to its cultural embeddedness and social acceptability. This was compounded by the cost and lack of availability of biomedical treatment, as highlighted by the service providers. The fact that 16 participants were not in formal employment and all participants did not have an adequate income to acquire services, attests the importance of socioeconomic status in treatment choice. Further, there was evidence that more educated participants had achieved greater mastery over their epilepsy than less educated participants. Though it was difficult to determine whether rural backgrounds had influenced participants' experiences in this study, it might be surmised that growing up in a rural area would predispose people with epilepsy to traditional treatments that were more prevalent in rural than urban populations in Africa because service quality was erratic (Watts, 1989, 1992). The over-reliance on traditional treatments was also linked to low economic status of participants since traditional treatment was more accessible than fee-based medical tests.

Effective strategies

Participants suggested several strategies to improve the employment of people with epilepsy. The strategies were informed by the biopsychosocial, social and human rights model of disability with limited focus on economic issues. They stressed the role of education, training, government and non-government services. However, their suggestions focused on services to individual on a case-by-case basis, though other suggestions highlighted the need for taking a structural approach. Another limitation of the suggestions was a neglect of the private sector. As suggested by the WHO (2016) and ILO (Hlatywayo et al., 2014; ILO, 2015), the private sector plays an important role in the delivery of employment services. The ILO (2015) recommended inclusion of awareness of disability issues to private sector employees. Hlatywayo et al. (2014) recommended incentives to the private sector to employ people with disability. The suggestions made by participants are discussed in turn.

Epilepsy education

Participants gave suggestions for epilepsy awareness, including borrowing from the HIV and AIDS model which was successfully used to end AIDS-related stigma. Epilepsy education was required to reduce stigma and to promote uptake or early medical treatment (Birbeck, 2000; Mushi et al., 2011; Watts, 1989; WHO, 2015). Literature showed that epilepsy stigma can be enacted and felt and could be experienced by families and co-workers too (Baskind & Birbeck, 2005a; Halima et al., 2017; Obeid, 2008). However, epilepsy stigma looks more complex than HIV-related stigma in that it is embedded in society as opposed to HIV stigma which was a new phenomenon. As this study showed, public awareness of epilepsy as a treatable condition increased treatment uptake, yet resources for nationwide awareness initiatives were non-existent, and government had not prioritised epilepsy in the allocation of public resources.

Government services

Government services focused on individual issues and did not take a structural approach. Even interview participants were more concerned with availability of social welfare grant and reserved jobs than policies to ensure sustainable social assistance and make government more accountable. Some service providers supported this direction. A missing suggestion was on having employment services provided by government to people with disability such as epilepsy yet literature shows this was important (Banks & Polack, 2015; Mhiribidi, 2010; Mitra, 2008; Mupedziswa, 2001; Mupedziswa & Kubanga, 2016). Failure to provide employment services for people with disability is not only costly to them and their families, but also their community and country (Banks & Polack, 2015; ILO, 2007, 2015). Though Zimbabwe has a strong infrastructure of public health services in urban areas, service quality is erratic, and hospitals are overcrowded and under-resourced. Reliable private services, though available, are expensive and out of the reach of most Zimbabweans. Lacking is a strong community health workforce educating communities about the ease with which epilepsy might be treated if properly understood as a neurological condition. The suggestion by service providers for government to fully implement international and regional protocols on disability were important.

Non-government services

A few of the participants like Sanga talked about representation of people with disability in policy-making structures such as parliament. While the ESF had joined the disability movement and had advocacy officers, its work was still lacking in this regard. Other groups of people with epilepsy were still not well represented, especially those in employment and those staying in rural communities. People with epilepsy in this study had received treatment and social support from the ESF in Harare, but most people living with epilepsy in Zimbabwe are severely disadvantaged by the prevalence of ignorance and the absence of appropriate resources, especially in rural areas (Duggan, 2013; Halima et al., 2017; Mushi et al., 2011; Nuhu et al., 2010). The dire economic situation in Zimbabwe did little to improve the situation.

The fact that the ESF had taken both a biopsychosocial model approach through the provision on health services and a social model through disability advocacy was commendable. The focus on epilepsy as a health condition, which is presently the dominant strategy in Zimbabwe, neglects the structural issues surrounding the condition, including the cultural impediments. Taking epilepsy as a disability is viable option, though once fully treated, it could cease to be a physical disability.

The viability rests in the point that Zimbabwe has a disability movement that has potential to advocate for better services, especially the removal of stigma. So, the disability option allows for structural impediments to social, economic and political advancement to be addressed wholesomely. But for epilepsy, medical treatment is crucial, hence a balance is required between medical and social goals.

Individual management

Participants recommended improving individual ability to manage epilepsy and to look for jobs. Despite the odds stacked against them, the findings showed that eight participants had demonstrated remarkable resilience by overcoming chronic unemployment. As pointed out by service providers, in the absence of reliable public services, people with epilepsy were left to self-manage their adversity. This confirms findings from other studies (Bradley et al., 2016; Day, 2008; Edward, Cook, & Giandinoto, 2015; Ring et al., 2016). Faced with numerous barriers, individual resilience acted as a strong coping mechanism that resulted in better employment outcomes for a few participants. Resilience was an individual psychological attribute but other individual factors like seizure type and age that impacted employment of people with epilepsy in several ways, but these were not fully explored in this study although the literature covered these extensively (Wo et al., 2016). These could be gaps for future research in Zimbabwe. However, relying on individual management was only a coping mechanism that should not stop service providers and service users from advocating for government-provided employment services to achieve social justice.

A major problem for people with epilepsy in Zimbabwe was their lack of representation in policy-making structures. People with epilepsy lacked a voice and concurred with service providers that a rights-based approach was needed to ensure social justice for people with epilepsy. Such an approach would enhance access to productive employment supported by policies and services to ensure fair treatment for, and prevent unfair dismissal of, people with epilepsy in the workplace. Representation would extend to policy-making structures within the workplace, as well as in broader policy networks. Recognition would guarantee social assistance for people with epilepsy to gain an education and access work, supported by accessible medical, health, education and social support services, in line with the ILO's (2007, 2015) recommendations on the employment of people with disability.

Conclusion

In conclusion, this chapter has highlighted the various challenges faced by people with epilepsy in resource-poor settings, using examples from a study conducted in Zimbabwe. It has examined how negative beliefs, inadequate public services, difficulties in job-seeking and issues with managing the condition impact their lives. Effective strategies to address these challenges include raising awareness to counteract harmful beliefs, improving public services, creating fair job opportunities and providing better support for self-management. The study's findings have significant implications for social policy and practice, guiding efforts to develop supportive systems and policies that enhance the well-being of people with epilepsy. With sustained effort at family, community, societal, continental and global levels, progress can be made towards a future where individuals with epilepsy in resource-poor settings receive the support they need to realise their capabilities.

References

Abidi, J., & Sharma, D. (2014). Poverty, disability, and employment: Global perspectives from the National Centre for Promotion of Employment for Disabled People. *Career Development for Exceptional Individuals, 37*(1), 60–68. doi:10.1177/2165143413520180

Adamolekun, B., Mielke, J. K., & Ball, D. E. (1999). An evaluation of the impact of health worker and patient education on the care and compliance of patients with epilepsy in Zimbabwe. *Epilepsia, 40,* 507–511. doi:10.1111/j.1528-1157.1999.tb00749.x

Al-Adawi, S., Al-Salmy, H., Martin, R. G., Al-Naamani, A., Prabhakar, S., Deleu, D., & Dorvlo, A. S. (2003). Patient's perspective on epilepsy: Self-knowledge among Omanis. *Seizure, 12*(1), 11–18.

Banks, L. M., & Polack, S. (2015). The economic costs of exclusion and gains of inclusion of people with disabilities. Evidence from low and middle income countries. Retrieved January 13, 2016 from https://disabilitycentre.lshtm.ac.uk/files/2014/07/Costs-of-Exclusion-and-Gains-of-Inclusion-Report.pdf

Baskind, R., & Birbeck, G. L. (2005a). Epilepsy care in Zambia: A study of traditional healers. *Epilepsia, 46*(7), 1121–1126. doi:10.1111/j.1528-1167.2005.03505.x

Birbeck, G. L. (2000). Seizures in rural Zambia. *Epilepsia, 41*(3), 277–281.

Bradley, P. M., Lindsay, B., & Fleeman, N. (2016). Care delivery and self management strategies for adults with epilepsy. *Cochrane Database of Systematic Review, 2.* doi:10.1002/14651858.CD006244.pub3

Buckup, S. (2009). *The price of exclusion: The economic consequences of excluding people with disabilities from the world of work.* ILO Employment Working Paper, 3. Geneva: ILO.

Chifamba, C. (2015). Being a Zimbabwean woman with a disability. *Her Zimbabwe Newspaper*, 11 June 2017.

Chitando, E., Gunda, M. R., & Kügler, J. (2013). Introduction. In E. Chitando, M. R. Gunda & J. Kügler (Eds.), *Prophets, profits and the Bible in Zimbabwe* (pp. 1–14). Bamberg: University of Bamberg Press.

Choruma, T. (2006). *The forgotten tribe: People with disabilities in Zimbabwe.* London: Progressio.

Coker, M. F., Bhargava, S., Fitzgerald, M., & Doherty, C. P. (2011). What do people with epilepsy know about their condition? Evaluation of a subspecialty clinic population. *Seizure, 20*(1), 55–59. doi:10.1016/j.seizure.2010.10.007

Cramm, J. M., Lorenzo, T., & Nieboer, A. P. (2014). Comparing education, employment, social support and well-being among youth with disabilities and their peers in South Africa. *Applied Research in Quality of Life, 9*(3), 517–524.

Cramm, J. M., Nieboer, A. P., Finkenflügel, H., & Lorenzo, T. (2013). Comparison of barriers to employment among youth with and without disabilities in South Africa. *Work, 46*(1), 19–24. doi:10.3233/WOR-121521

Danermark, B., & Coniavitis, L. G. (2004). Social justice: Redistribution and recognition-a non-reductionist perspective on disability. *Disability and Society, 19*(4), 339–353.

Day, K. (2008). *Quality of life: The role of psychological resilience.* Thesis-Clinical Psychology Document Number 155. University of Edinburgh, Edinburgh.

Dewa, E., January, J., Nyati-Jokomo, Z., Mafaune, P. T., Muteti, S., & Maradzika, J. (2014). Non-attendance of treatment review visits among epileptic patients in a rural district, Zimbabwe. *Journal of Public Health in Africa, 5*(2), 73–76. doi:10.4081/jphia.2014.351

Dube, L., Shoko, T., & Haves, S. (2011). *African initiatives in healing ministry.* Pretoria: Unisa Press.

Duggan, M. B. (2013). Epilepsy and its effects on children and families in rural Uganda. *African Health Sciences, 13*(3), 613–623. doi:10.4314/ahs.v13i3.14

Échevin, D. (2013). Employment and education discrimination against disabled people in Cape Verde. *Applied Economics, 45*(7), 857–875. doi:10.1080/00036846.2011.613775

Edward, K., Cook, M., & Giandinoto, J. (2015). An integrative review of the benefits of self-management interventions for adults with epilepsy. *Epilepsy & Behavior, 45,* 195–204.

Elger, C. E., & Schmidt, D. (2008). Modern management of epilepsy: A practical approach. *Epilepsy & Behavior, 12*(4), 501–539. doi:10.1016/j.yebeh.2008.01.003

Elliott, J., & Shneker, B. (2008). Patient, caregiver, and health care practitioner knowledge of, beliefs about, and attitudes toward epilepsy. *Epilepsy & Behavior, 12*(4), 547–556. doi:10.1016/j.yebeh.2007.11.008

Erickson, W. A., von Schrader, S., Bruyère, S. M., & VanLooy, S. A. (2014). The employment environment: Employer perspectives, policies, and practices regarding the employment of persons with disabilities. *Rehabilitation Counseling Bulletin, 57*(4), 195–208. doi:10.1177/0034355213509841

Foundation for Scientific and Industrial Research at the Norwegian Institute of Technology (SINTEF). (2003). *Living conditions among people with activity limitations in Zimbabwe: A representative regional study.* Harare: SINTEF.

Fraser, N. (2001). *Social justice in the knowledge society: Redistribution, recognition and participation.* Berlin: Heinrich Boll Stiftung.

Gathiram, N. (2008). A critical review of the developmental approach to disability in South Africa. *International Journal of Social Welfare, 17*(2), 146–155. doi:10.1111/j.1468-2397.2007.00551.x

Government of Zimbabwe. (1988). *Social Welfare Assistance Act.* Harare: Government of Zimbabwe.

Government of Zimbabwe. (1992). *Disabled Persons Act.* Harare: Government of Zimbabwe.

Government of Zimbabwe. (2005). *Labour Act.* Harare: Government of Zimbabwe.

Government of Zimbabwe. (2011). *Country report on human rights of persons with disabilities.* Geneva: Mission of the Republic of Zimbabwe to the Office of the United Nations.

Government of Zimbabwe. (2012). *Zimbabwe population census report.* Harare: Government of Zimbabwe.

Halima, F. S. N., Ndiaye, M., Magnerou, A. M., Hamza, H., Sow, A. D., & Ndiaye, M. M. (2017). *Lives of people with epilepsy at work in Dakar.* Paper presented at the 3rd African Epilepsy Congress, Dakar Senegal, May 5–7, 2017.

Hlatywayo, L., Hlatywayo, S., & Mtezo, J. Z. (2014). The employment of deaf persons: A Zimbabwean employers perspective. *Journal of Humanities and Social Science, 19*(9), 37–42.

Honneth, A. (1997). Recognition and moral obligation. *Social Research, 64*(1), 16–35.

Hounsossou, C. H., Queneuille, J. P., Ibinga, E., Preux, P. M., Dalmay, F., Druet-Cabanac, M., & Houinato, D. (2015). Knowledge, attitudes, and behavior among key people involved in the employment of people with epilepsy in southern Benin. *Epilepsy & Behavior, 42*, 153–158. doi:10.1016/j.yebeh.2014.10.022.

International Labour Organisation (ILO). (2001). *Code of practice for managing disability in the workplace.* Retrieved March 12, 2016 from https://www.ilo.org/public/english/standards/relm/gb/docs/gb282/pdf/tmemdw-2.pdf

International Labour Organisation (ILO). (2007). *Skills development through community based rehabilitation (CBR). A good practice guide.* Geneva: ILO.

International Labour Organisation (ILO). (2015). *Disability inclusion strategy and action plan 2014–2017.* Retrieved October 1, 2016 from https://www.ilo.org/global/topics/disability-and-work/WCMS_475650/lang--en/index.htm

International Labour Organisation (ILO). (2016). *Decent work and the 2030 Agenda for sustainable development.* Retrieved October 13, 2016 from https://www.ilo.org/global/topics/sdg-2030/lang--en/index.htm

International Labour Organisation (ILO). (2017). *Disability and work.* Retrieved January 26, 2017 from https://ilo.org/global/topics/disability-and-work/WCMS_475650/lang--en/index.html

International League Against Epilepsy (ILAE), World Health Organisation (WHO), & International Bureau for Epilepsy (IBE). (2000). *African Declaration on Epilepsy.* Dakar: Senegal.

Jackson, H., & Mupedziswa, R. (1988). Disability and rehabilitation: Beliefs and attitudes among rural disabled people in a community based rehabilitation scheme in Zimbabwe. *Journal of Social Development in Africa, 3*(1), 21–30.

Jacoby, A., & Baker, G. A. (2008). Quality-of-life trajectories in epilepsy: A review of the literature. *Epilepsy & Behavior, 12*(4), 557–571. doi:10.1016/j.yebeh.2007.11.013

Jacoby, A., Gorry, J., & Baker, G. A. (2005). Employers' attitudes to employment of people with epilepsy: Still the same old story? *Epilepsia (Series 4), 46*(12), 1978–1987. doi:10.1111/j.1528-1167.2005.00345.x

Kazembe, T. (2009). The relationship between God and people in Shona Traditional Religion. *The Rose+Croix Journal, 6*, 51–79.

Keikelame, M. J., & Swartz, L. (2015). 'A thing full of stories': Traditional healers' explanations of epilepsy and perspectives on collaboration with biomedical health care in Cape Town. *Transcultural Psychiatry, 52*(5), 659–680. doi:10.1177/1363461515571626

Knight, A. (2015). Democratizing disability: Achieving inclusion (without assimilation) through "Participatory Parity". *Hypatia, 30*(1), 97–114. doi:10.1111/hypa.12120

Lang, R., & Charowa, G. (2007). Disability scoping study in Zimbabwe: Final report. Harare: DFID.

Liao, J., & Zhao, J. (2013). *Rate of returns to education of persons with disabilities in rural China.* Paper presented at the International Conference on Applied Social Science Research (ICASSR), Shanghai, China, June 2013. doi:10.2991/icassr.2013.60

Madzokere, C. (1997). Life experiences of people with epilepsy. A study of Highfield high density residential area in Harare, Zimbabwe. *EPICADEC News (Biannual Newsletter of Foundation Epilepsy Care Developing Countries), 10*(97), 19–21.

Magazi, D. (2017). *The role of traditional healers in the ongoing management of epilepsy.* Paper presented at the 3rd African Epilepsy Congress, Dakar Senegal, May 5–7, 2017.

Maja, P. A., Mann, W. M., Sing, D., Steyn, A. J., & Naidoo, P. (2011). Employing people with disabilities in South Africa. *South African Journal of Occupational Therapy, 41*(1), 24–32.

Marongwe, N., & Mate, R. (2007). *Children with disability: Their households' livelihoods and experiences in accessing key services.* Harare: United Nations Food and Agriculture Organisation.

Marumoagae, M. C. (2012). Disability discrimination and the right of disabled persons to access the labour market. *Potchefstroom Electronic Law Journal, 15*(1), 244–365. doi:10.4314/pelj.v15i1.10

McNay, L. (2008). The trouble with recognition: Subjectivity, suffering, and agency. *Sociological Theory, 26*(3), 271–296. doi:10.1111/j.1467-9558.2008.00329.x

Meinardi, H., Scott, R. A., Reis, R., & Sander, J. W. (2001). The treatment gap in epilepsy: The current situation and ways forward. *Epilepsia, 42*(1), 136–149.

Mhiribidi, S. T. W. (2010). Promoting the developmental social welfare approach in Zimbabwe: Challenges and prospects. *Journal of Social Development in Africa, 25*(2), 121–146.

Mielke, J., Adamolekun, B., Ball, D., & Mundanda, T. (1997). Knowledge and attitudes of teachers towards epilepsy in Zimbabwe. *Acta Neurologica Scandinavica, 96*(3), 133–137.

Mitra, S. (2008). The recent decline in the employment of persons with disabilities in South Africa, 1998–2006. *South African Journal of Economics, 76*(3), 480–492. doi:10.1111/j.1813-6982.2008.00196.x

Mizunoya, S., & Mitra, S. (2013). Is there a disability gap in employment rates in developing countries? *World Development, 42*, 28–43. doi:10.1016/j.worlddev.2012.05.037

Mtetwa, E. (2011). Policy dimensions of exclusion: Disability as charity and not right in Zimbabwe. *Indian Journal of Social Work, 72*(3), 381–398.

Mugumbate, J., & Mushonga, J. (2013). Myths, perceptions, and incorrect knowledge surrounding epilepsy in rural Zimbabwe: A study of the villagers in Buhera District. *Epilepsy & Behavior, 27*(1), 144–147. doi:10.1016/j.yebeh.2012.12.036

Mugumbate, J., & Nyanguru, A. (2013). Measuring the challenges of people with epilepsy in Harare, Zimbabwe. *Neurology Asia, 18*(1), 29–33.

Munn, Z. (2008). Care delivery and self-management strategies for adults with epilepsy. *Journal of Advanced Nursing, 64*, 455–456.

Mupedziswa, R. (2001). The quest for relevance: Towards a conceptual model of developmental social work education and training in Africa. *International Social Work, 44*(3), 285–300.

Mupedziswa, R., & Kubanga, K. (2016). Developing social work education in Africa: Challenges and prospects. In I. Taylor, M. Bogo, M. Lefevre, & B. Teater (Eds.), *Routledge international handbook of social work education* (pp. 119–130). London: Routledge.

Mushi, D., Hunter, E., Mtuya, C., Mshana, G., Aris, E., & Walker, R. (2011). Social-cultural aspects of epilepsy in Kilimanjaro Region, Tanzania: Knowledge and experience among patients and carers. *Epilepsy and Behaviour, 20*, 338–343.

Mutanana, N., & Mutara, G. (2015). Health seeking behaviours of people with epilepsy in a rural community of Zimbabwe. *International Journal of Research in Humanities and Social Studies, 2*(2), 87–96.

Nuhu, F. T., Fawole, J. O., Babalola, O. J., Ayilara, O. O., & Sulaiman, Z. T. (2010). Social consequences of epilepsy: A study of 231 Nigerian patients. *Annals of African Medicine, 9*(3), 170–175. doi: 10.4103/1596-3519.68360

Obeid, T. (2008). Stigma: An aspect of epilepsy not to be ignored. *Saudi Medical Journal, 29*(4), 489–497.

Peta, C., McKenzie, J., & Kathard, H. (2015). Voices from the periphery: A narrative study of the experiences of sexuality of disabled women in Zimbabwe. *Agenda, 29*(2), 66–76. doi:10.1080/10130950.2015.1050783

Richardson, C. E. (2002). The metatheory of resilience and resiliency. *Journal of Clinical Psychology, 58*(3), 307–321.

Ring, A., Jacob, A., Baker, G., Marson, A., & Whitehead, M. (2016). Does the concept of resilience contribute to understanding good quality of life in the context of epilepsy? *Epilepsy & Behavior, 56*, 153–164.

Saburi, G., Mapanga, K. G., & Mapanga, M. B. (2006). Perceived family reactions and quality of life of adults with epilepsy. *Neuroscience Nursing, 38*(3), 156.

Schneider, M., Mokomane, Z., & Graham, L. (2016). Social protection, chronic poverty and disability: Applying an intersectionality perspective. In S. Grech & K. Soldatic (Eds.), *Disability in the global south: The critical handbook* (pp. 365–376). Gewerbstrasse: Springer.

Schur, L., Kruse, D., Blasi, J., & Blanck, P. (2009). Is disability disabling in all workplaces? Workplace disparities and corporate culture. *Industrial Relations, 48*(3), 381–410. doi:10.1111/j.1468-232X.2009.00565.x

Sebit, M. B., & Mielke, J. (2005). Epilepsy in Sub-Saharan Africa: Its socio-demography, aetiology, diagnosis and EEG characteristics in Harare, Zimbabwe. *East African Medical Journal, 82*(3), 128–137.

Soeker, M. S., Van Rensburg, V., & Travill, A. (2012). Individuals with traumatic brain injuries perceptions and experiences of returning to work in South Africa. *Work, 42*(4), 589–600.

Sung, C., Muller, V., Jones, J. E., & Fong, C. (2014). Vocational rehabilitation service patterns and employment outcomes of people with epilepsy. *Epilepsy Research, 108*(8), 1469–1479. doi:10.1016/j.eplepsyres.2014.06.016

Tai, S. (2011). Social and psychological issues in patients with epilepsy. In H. Foyaca-Sibat (Ed.), *Novel aspects on epilepsy* (pp. 67–88). Rijeka: InTech.

Transparency International Zimbabwe. (2015). *Annual state of corruption report: Focus on state-owned enterprises.* Harare: Transparency International Zimbabwe.

van Niekerk, L. (2010). Disability stereotypes defied by life stories. *South African Journal of Occupational Therapy, 40*(S), 15–22.

Watts, A. E. (1989). A model for managing epilepsy in a rural community in Africa. *British Medical Journal, 298*, 235–268. doi:10.1136/bmj.298.6676.805

Watts, A. E. (1992). The natural history of untreated epilepsy in a rural community in Africa. *Epilepsia, 33*(3), 464–468.

Wiggett-Barnard, C., & Swartz, L. (2012). What facilitates the entry of persons with disabilities into South African companies? *Disability & Rehabilitation, 34*(12), 1016–1023.

Winkler, A. S., Mayer, M., Ombay, M., Mathias, B., Schmutzhard, E., & Jilek-Aall, L. (2009). Attitudes towards African traditional medicine and Christian spiritual healing regarding treatment of epilepsy in a rural community of northern Tanzania. *African Journal Traditional Complementary Alternative Medicine, 7*(2), 162–170.

Wo, M. M., Lim, K. S., Choo, W. Y., & Tan, C. T. (2016). Factors affecting the employability in people with epilepsy. *Epilepsy Research, 1286*, 11. doi:10.1016/j.eplepsyres.2016.10.003

Wolffe, K. E., Ajuwon, P. M., & Kelly, S. M. (2013a). Working with visual impairment in Nigeria: A qualitative look at employment status. *Journal of Visual Impairment & Blindness, 107*(6), 425–436.

World Health Organisation (WHO). (2015). *Sixty-Eighth World Health Assembly adopts resolution on epilepsy.* Geneva: WHO.
World Health Organisation (WHO). (2016). *Epilepsy.* Retrieved October 16, 2016 from https://www.who.int/mediacentre/factsheets/fs999/en/
Yuh, J., Yun-Tung, W., Meng-Hsiu, L., & Shih, K. J. (2013). Predictors of employment outcomes for people with visual impairment in Taiwan: The contribution of disability employment services. *Journal of Visual Impairment & Blindness, 107*(6), 469–480.

7 The employment challenge in detail

Employment is a type of livelihood. Livelihoods are ways of getting resources required to meet needs while income refers to the resources obtained from livelihoods. Livelihoods can include working in the productive or primary sectors, such as farming, fishing and mining or in services or secondary sectors, such as education, retail, administration and marketing. For people with epilepsy, income is usually not there, or is inadequate due to low education and training but also social conditions that prevent them from participating equally in society. Most end up in self-employment or having to rely on government social assistance. This chapter furthers the issues of employment raised in the previous chapter using 15 case studies from Zimbabwe. These 15 were young people with epilepsy who had different experiences with employment. The common themes from these experiences will be discussed. To deepen the discussion, service-user perspectives will be shared and discussed and lessons for other human service professionals shared.

The concepts of livelihoods, income and employment

In a livelihood, there is a person who engages in an activity to gain income, which can be either monetary or non-monetary (International Labour Organisation [ILO], 2005a, 2005b). This actor may work in various sectors, such as farming, fishing or services, to obtain the resources they need. The activities they undertake are essential for supporting their daily needs and improving their overall well-being, and non-monetary income can include goods or services received in exchange for work, such as bartering or subsistence activities.

Income is the money or things a person earns or receives. It can come from different places, like a job, business or investments. For farmers, income can come from selling crops, livestock, or other products they produce. In countries like Vietnam and Chile, growing crops is an important source of income, as farmers sell rice, fruits and vegetables. In mining, income is earned from extracting and selling minerals, while in fisheries, income comes from catching and selling fish or other seafood. In Senegal and Malawi, fishing is a crucial source of income, providing livelihoods for many families. People can have formal jobs, which are regular and often come with benefits, or informal jobs, which are less secure and may not have official contracts. In places like Bali and Guyana, tourism is also an important

DOI: 10.4324/9781003602866-7

source of income for families, as they earn money by providing services to visitors, such as accommodation, food and guided tours. This income is important because it helps people buy what they need, like food and housing. It can come regularly, like a salary, or from time to time, like a bonus or gift.

The term employment, and its affiliates work, job, labour market or economic participation, and livelihood, as defined by the ILO (2007), does not necessarily refer to formal paid work, but also includes informal unpaid or self-help jobs, unpaid domestic work and individual businesses or microenterprises. The ILO has long distinguished between paid work and self-employment (or informal work) (ILO, 1993) seeing both as important for economic empowerment (ILO, 2007). Paid employment involves oral or verbal contracts and a basic income (salary or wage or, at times, commissions and bonuses), or in-kind payments not dependent on the revenue of the employer, and self-employment work, where remuneration accrues from profits from the sale of goods or services (ILO, 1993). The ILO (1993) defined employed people as:

> Persons who during a specified brief period such as one week or one day, (a) performed some work for wage or salary in cash or in kind, (b) had a formal attachment to their job but were temporarily not at work during the reference period, (c) performed some work for profit or family gain in cash or in kind, (d) were with an enterprise such as a business, farm or service but who were temporarily not at work during the reference period for any specific reason.
>
> (p. 47)

The ILO (2016) argues for 'decent work' in the formal and informal economies, that is, work that enables people to survive and develop, and live quality lives. Decent work affords people a minimal wage of more than US$2 a day and can lift people out of poverty (ILO, 2016). For many people, however, work is anything but decent. It pays a meagre income for those for whom poverty continues unabated. The SDGs seek to increase the number of jobs and promote decent work by 2030 (United Nations [UN], 2015). SDG8 aims to 'promote sustained, inclusive and sustainable economic growth, full and productive employment and decent work for all' (UN, 2015, para. 1).

Epilepsy and employment globally

Despite laws prohibiting workplace discrimination, people with disabilities of working age often find themselves unable to acquire and maintain jobs leading to socioeconomic loss for individuals, families, communities, businesses and nations (ILO, 2013, 2017). Based on research from ten low- and middle-income countries, including Zimbabwe, the ILO (2015) estimated that the economic cost of disability exclusion was between 3% and 7% of the Gross Domestic Product (GDP) worldwide. This form of injustice contributed to poverty among people with disabilities and represented a huge socioeconomic loss that could not be ignored (ILO, 2017).

To address this injustice, studies were needed to highlight the factors preventing the economic participation of people with disabilities like epilepsy. A review of literature relating to epilepsy and employment outside Africa revealed several themes as follows: (i) individual predictors of employment outcomes, (ii) social barriers to employment and (iii) role of employment services. These themes are discussed in turn while literature from African studies was discussed in the subsequent section because it was few.

Individual predictors of employment outcomes

Researchers have tried to understand individual factors associated with employment outcomes among people with epilepsy. More recent research on predictors of employment among 146 people with epilepsy in Malaysia reported that high employability related to high self-esteem, high self-determined motivation, low self-perceived stigma and availability of social support. Of the participants, 64.4% achieved high employability. Other factors that necessitated employability were education, type of epilepsy, ability to cope, lower family expectations and overprotection. People with generalised seizures were found to have better employment outcomes (Wo et al., 2015). The researchers proposed an employment model with three elements: (i) assessment of ability to work and provision of appropriate training, (ii) identifying positive factors in family and workplace and (iii) cultivating self-determined motivation. An earlier systematic review by Wo, Lim, Choo and Tan (2015) found that the adjusted employment rate of people with uncontrolled seizures was comparable to those with controlled seizures. This result showed that factors that influenced employment were not only clinical but also social. While this study, and other discussed below provided insights into employment issues, they focused on demographic, clinical and psychological factors and not systemic factors (Wo et al., 2015).

A longitudinal study in Finland followed participants who were younger than 16 years until they reached 48 years of age (n = 119) (Sillanpää & Schmidt, 2010). The study found that later onset of epilepsy in children of normal intelligence (i.e., occurring at the age of six years or older) was a reliable predictor of employment in early adulthood, especially with good vocational education. Normal intelligence, having offspring, uninterrupted remission, and no history of status epilepticus (a continuous seizure that is dangerous for a person with epilepsy) appeared to predict lasting employment into midlife (Sillanpää & Schmidt, 2010). The three most significant factors were normal intelligence, age at diagnosis of epilepsy older than six years, and vocational education (at age 23 years). At 48 years, no history of status epilepticus and normal intelligence were the most significant factors. Even without intellectual handicap, Sillanpää and Schmidt (2010) found that the long-term employment outcome appeared unsatisfactory in adults with childhood-onset epilepsy, findings supported by Geerts et al. (2011) Netherlands study. Nevertheless, in the Finnish study by Sillanpää and Schmidt (2010), about 60% of respondents with childhood-onset epilepsy had entered employment as adults. The unemployment rate was significantly higher throughout the follow-up period among the epilepsy sample than in the general population in the study area: at 23 and 48 years of age, respectively, the unemployment rate was 4.9% (in 1982) and 6.2% (in 2007). Other studies confirm the impact on severity of seizures in Korea, respectively (Sang-Ahm, 2005). More epilepsy awareness was recommended.

Individual psychosocial functioning was associated with better employment outcomes. This was shown by Smeets, van Lierop, Vanhoutvin, Aldenkamp and Nijhuis (2007) who reviewed 24 studies on epilepsy and employment and concluded that there were complex interacting problems affecting employment, such as stigma, seizure severity and psychological variables, such as low self-esteem, passive coping style and low self-efficacy. They recommended specific training interventions to improve self-efficacy and coping skills. Their conclusions and recommended strategies focused on the individual person with epilepsy whom they expected to 'accept their disorder and make personal and health-related choices that help them to achieve better employment positions in society' (Smeets et al., 2007, p. 354).

Research showed that people with epilepsy were affected by individual factors differently since they were not a homogenous group but varied by age, gender, type of epilepsy, social class and other variables (Holland, Lane, Whitehead, Marson, & Jacoby, 2009). To understand differences that emanated from some of these variables, Holland et al. (2009) studied 350 individuals with epilepsy who were of working age. They examined labour market participation following the onset of seizures and early epilepsy. Employment rates were calculated for the cohort and general population. Employment trajectories over four years were explored in terms of occupational social class. The relative risk of employment was calculated by clinical features of seizures and social class. People who had recently experienced a single seizure or who had early onset epilepsy experienced substantial employment disadvantages. Holland et al. (2009) recommended that greater efforts were needed to help these people return to work and stay employed.

Social barriers in the workplace

While researchers cited in the preceding section dwelt on individual factors, others such as Bishop (2002) focused on social barriers to employment. A study in the USA by Bishop (2002) found that for a person with epilepsy, attaining employment often involved the negotiation of numerous obstacles, including navigating the relationship between work, epilepsy and its treatment, often in the context of negative and uninformed attitudes and beliefs of employers and co-workers. These results underscored the complexity of the process of seeking, attaining and maintaining work for a person with epilepsy. Bishop (2002) found that barriers included employers' fear of elevated accident rates, increased insurance rates and concerns about workers' safety. Likewise, a study of 204 employers in the UK concluded that epilepsy created high rates of concern for 50% of employers, especially relating to the likelihood of work-related accidents (Jacoby, Gorry, & Baker, 2005). In

Bishop's (2002) study, in discussing the disclosure of his epilepsy to his employer, one discussant said:

> Every job I have, as soon as they find out, there are excuses and excuses and reasons to throw me out the door. And really there is nothing that I cannot accomplish or that I cannot do. Give me a few minutes if I have an aura or if I have a simple seizure, it's not a big deal.
>
> (p. 284)

The challenges highlighted were social in nature and related to employer attitudes, as reported in other studies. In a study of employers (n = 204) across 14 employment sectors in the UK, Jacoby et al. (2005) reported that employment was one area of quality of life known to be compromised by epilepsy and that employer attitudes contributed to the employment problems of people with epilepsy. Twenty-six percent of respondents reported having experience of employing people with epilepsy; 16% considered that there were no jobs in their company suitable for people with epilepsy; 21% thought employing people with epilepsy would be 'a major issue'. Employers were uniformly of the view that people with epilepsy, even when in remission, should disclose their condition to a prospective employer. Seizure severity, frequency and controllability were all considered important features of epilepsy in the employment context, reported Jacoby et al. (2005). Attitudes to employment of people with epilepsy were influenced by company size and type, and previous experience. However, it is worth noting that, in Jacoby et al.'s (2005) study, employers were willing to accommodate people with epilepsy, through job sharing, temporary reassignment of duties and flexible working hours. Similar sentiments were found in the review of literature on disability and employment (Erickson, von Schrader, Bruyère, & VanLooy, 2014; Jacoby & Baker, 2008; Ju, Roberts, & Zhang, 2013).

Discriminatory experiences

In South Korea, Sang-Ahm (2005) studied the employability of 543 people with epilepsy and found several barriers to employment that resulted in 31% unemployment for people with epilepsy, five times more than the general population. Participants reported that they were not given jobs once their condition was known. In Malaysia, Lim, Wo, Wong and Tan (2013) studied 250 people with epilepsy and found that gender and education impacted on employment opportunities, despite a strong economy; those who were employed were in part-time or low-paid employment.

Employment services

Sung, Muller, Jones and Fong's (2014) study on vocational rehabilitation service patterns and employment outcomes of previously unemployed people with epilepsy, who had received services (n = 2,030), found 884 (43.5%) achieved successful competitive employment. Their results indicated that higher education levels and accessible vocational rehabilitation services were positively related to successful employment outcomes. In contrast, Sung et al. (2014) reported having co-occurring anxiety and depression, receiving cash benefits or a prolonged period in the vocational rehabilitation system was negatively associated with employment. Other specific vocational rehabilitation services (e.g., education, vocational training and job search and placement assistance) were also found to be significant predictors of employment. Services provided by state vocational rehabilitation agencies were proven to be beneficial in improving employment outcomes. People with epilepsy were encouraged to pursue vocational rehabilitation services to increase their chances of attaining employment (Edward, Cook, & Giandinoto, 2015; Sung et al., 2014). Sung et al. (2014) reported that employment services were helpful to improve the acquisition of work skills, make job-seeking productive and ensure employees with disabilities could work productively and retain their positions.

Role of self-management and resilience

Dealing with the economic, social, political, cultural, biomedical and psychological problems brought by epilepsy required self-management abilities from the individual (Day, 2008; Edward et al., 2015; Ring, Jacob, Baker, Marson, & Whitehead, 2016; Taylor et al., 2011). Self-management included adaptive behaviours that a person used to control seizures including compliance with treatment, safety (e.g., stop driving) and other activities aimed at reducing triggers, argued Day (2008). Al-Adawi et al. (2003) found that knowledge of epilepsy increased a mastery of epilepsy and this reduced challenges for people with epilepsy. However, people with epilepsy did not always have correct and adequate knowledge about their condition (Al-Adawi et al., 2003; Coker, Bhargava, Fitzgerald, & Doherty, 2011). Resilient individuals had the potential to 'recover, adjust, resist stress and potentially thrive in the face of adversity' (Edward et al., 2015, p. 196). Psychological resilience was the ability to adapt to stressful events with good outcomes (Day, 2008). Studies by Day (2008) and Edward et al. (2015) downplayed the role of seizure frequency in quality of life and argued that resilience was more pronounced. Taylor et al. (2011) reached the same conclusion in their examination of adults with epilepsy.

Self-management was found to play a positive role in the lives of people with epilepsy supported by educational and lifestyle management programmes. A study by Munn (2008) found that self-management education improved the knowledge and self-confidence of adults. They were better able to deal with psychological stressors and reported better seizure control and quality of life and they had better knowledge of symptoms (Jacoby & Baker, 2008; Munn, 2008). Munn (2008) recommended the use of individualised approaches to deal with the multiple challenges of people with epilepsy, such as those shown in Table 7.1.

Table 7.1 Techniques to foster self-management and resilience

Category	Technique
Individual factors	Self-esteem
	Vocational education
	Positive adjustment to diagnosis of epilepsy
	Social life skills
	Knowledge of epilepsy
Environmental factors	Early treatment
	Positive family environment
	Counselling
	Peer involvement and support
	Psychosocial education and behavioural interventions
	Epilepsy and health education

Richardson's (2002) resiliency model presumed that, faced with adversities, like epilepsy, individuals experienced biopsychosocial disruption, after which they reintegrated in a manner that improved their resilience and reduced their vulnerability. Self-management increased coping, understanding, treatment adherence and seizure control, all of which were important for employment (Lindsay & Fleeman, 2016; Munn, 2008).

African studies

There was little information from Africa on epilepsy and employment. Only two articles focused on employment directly (Halima et al., 2017; Hounsossou et al., 2015). Three addressed employment in passing (Mushi et al., 2011; Nuhu, Fawole, Babalola, Ayilara, & Sulaiman, 2010; Obiako et al., 2014), while 11 dealt with issues of treatment and education.

Halima et al. (2017) studied discrimination in Senegal. Forms of discrimination reported by two-thirds of participants included job degradation, lack of promotion and the threat of dismissal. Most (98%) people with epilepsy who participated in the study worked in the tertiary industries. Most (78%) had disclosed their condition to their employers. Twenty-four (56%) reported that work impacted on their epilepsy, while 84% reported that epilepsy impacted on their work. The researchers concluded that there was a relationship between epilepsy (seizures in the workplace) and work (stress-inducing work environments).

Hounsossou et al. (2015) found negative attitudes towards people with epilepsy in Benin, despite the fact that participants had a fairly accurate understanding of epilepsy (95.3% supported mainstream education for people with epilepsy). For example, only 28.6% of respondents said they would employ a person with epilepsy, while 25% said epilepsy was contagious. However, the study did not include people with epilepsy.

Nuhu et al. (2010) found negative attitudes towards people with epilepsy and consequent social difficulties. Likewise, Mushi et al. (2011) found that people with epilepsy faced socioeconomic exclusion exacerbated by misunderstandings about epilepsy. These researchers recommended epilepsy awareness and improved treatment.

Obiako et al.'s (2014) study of 242 people with epilepsy in Nigeria found that there were limited education and employment opportunities for them: 50% had not finished school, 73% had no jobs, while 5% reported negative attitudes from employers and co-workers. They called for more awareness and psychosocial support interventions like counselling. Soumaila et al.'s (2017) survey of teachers in Niger found they held negative beliefs about epilepsy, believing it was contagious and incurable, even with modern medicine. Similarly, Morenikeji et al. (2017) found that 7% of the teachers they surveyed in Nigeria believed that children with epilepsy should not attend school. In Uganda, Duggan (2013) found that children with epilepsy and their families encountered stigma and discrimination resulting in low school attendance. Only 92 of the 162 school-aged children in the study were attending school. Likwise, Quereshi et al.'s (2017) Tanzanian study found that children's learning difficulties emanated from the stigma and poor educational support.

Doumbe, Bikek, Kuate and Njamnsh (2017) found that a significant number of health workers in Cameroon had incorrect knowledge of, and negative attitudes towards, people with epilepsy and some failed to treat them properly. In Guinea, Balde, Cisse, Toure, Kouyate and Balde (2017) found that a significant number of people with epilepsy preferred traditional treatments because they were cheaper though they often mixed biomedical and traditional treatments resulting in prolonged periods of seizures. Similar findings were reported in Tanzania (Mushi et al., 2011; Quereshi et al., 2017; Winkler et al., 2009). In Togo, Assogba, Waklasti, Kombate, Apetse and Balogou (2017) found 132 people with epilepsy had low adherence to treatment due to a lack of correct information about epilepsy. This was compounded by treatment personnel's ignorance about appropriate interventions.

Individual functioning was reported in three quality of life studies for people with epilepsy (Madzokere, 1997; Mielke, Sebit, & Adamolekun, 2000; Saburi, Mapanga, & Mapanga, 2006). Madzokere (1997) found high levels of stigma among people with epilepsy though women with epilepsy were more disadvantaged. Mielke et al. (2000) found that 36 of the 38 people with epilepsy in their sample and their carers did not believe that their epilepsy interfered with their social functioning, work performance, or relationships with others. Saburi et al. (2006) reported fear, isolation and secrecy. Mugumbate and Nyanguru (2013) measured the challenges of 60 people with epilepsy in Harare and found most were psychosocial, followed by economic and lifestyle. The most common issues were: securing an adequate income (93%), standard of living (83%), and finding and maintaining employment (78%). Related to these challenges was limited education among people with epilepsy. Saburi (2011) noted that children with epilepsy did not attend school or their attendance was poor. Families were not giving adequate support to their family members with epilepsy, especially educational support.

Social challenges were reported in a study by Vyas, Wong, Yang, Thistle and Lee (2016). The study found that stigma was a major challenge for people with epilepsy, who were often misunderstood as demon possessed. Socioeconomic challenges were linked to myths, misunderstandings and incorrect knowledge about epilepsy (Mugumbate & Mushonga, 2013). Myths, such as the notion that epilepsy was contagious, restricted association with people with epilepsy. Where such misunderstanding existed, even for employers who were part of this community, employing a person with epilepsy was problematic. Mielke, Adamolekun, Ball and Mundanda (1997) reported that 55.5% of 165 teachers surveyed in a peri-urban area near Harare said they would employ a person with epilepsy; 82% said they would allow their child to play with an epileptic child; 76% would marry an 'epileptic'; 22.6% thought that epilepsy was contagious; 12.6% thought it was a form of insanity; and 0.6% thought it was caused by evil spirits. However, their sample comprised educated people who were generally positive towards people with epilepsy. Misunderstanding was also reported by Butau and Piachaud (1993) who found a lack of correct knowledge among parents of children with epilepsy and Dewa et al. (2014) reported high levels of stigma in Zimbabwe.

Poor access to health services was reported in other studies. For example, Manungo (1993) found that Zimbabwe's health delivery system was inaccessible, resulting in people failing to comply with epilepsy treatment. Health centres were few and far between and drugs were often in short supply. Ball, Mielke, Adamolekun, Mundanda and McLean (2000) reported similar findings and recommended primary healthcare, health education, training of health personnel in epilepsy management, and increased supply of medicines, especially first-line medicines. Mielke (2006) recommended the supply of first-choice drugs, such as phenobarbital, because of their low cost and the training of primary care nurses to compensate for the shortage of doctors. Other studies focused on the quality of healthcare and found that therapeutic drug monitoring was essential to determine whether people with epilepsy were properly medicated and taking their medication (Ball & Taderera, 2003; Nhachi & Mwaluko, 1990). Adamolekun, Levy, Mielke and Zhande (1996) found out that EEG services were expensive but useful in confirming seizure types, thereby improving treatment. Dewa et al. (2014) found that people with epilepsy missed treatment due to a shortage of medicines and the distance they needed to travel to access health services. Birbeck (2008) highlighted the scarcity of specialist epilepsy services in Zimbabwe. Sebit and Mielke (2005) found that one in five people with epilepsy used traditional treatments first and the same number had gone back to traditional healers following biomedical treatment due to a lack of proper health education and services. Resultantly, medical treatment was delayed or ceased leading to more complex seizures and traditional treatments contributed to reduced opportunities for people with epilepsy.

Conclusion

This chapter reviewed the literature on disability, epilepsy and employment globally before reviewing literature on epilepsy and employment in Africa including Zimbabwe. Methodologically, reviewed studies were diverse, including both quantitative, qualitative and mixed methods. However, like this study, most were urban focused. The literature review showed that globally people with disability such as epilepsy were likely to face exclusion in education, employment, health and participation in the community due to attitudinal and policy barriers. The same situation pertained in Zimbabwe and many other African countries. The review identified some gaps in the literature. First, there is a dearth of literature on epilepsy and employment in Africa including Zimbabwe. Literature available in Zimbabwe was predominantly health focused and did not adequately deal with economic and structural dynamics that sustained stigma and discrimination. Second, there were very few social work studies with non-specific to employment issues in Africa and Zimbabwe. Nevertheless, the literature provided an understanding of the management of epilepsy. The next chapter provides more information on Zimbabwe with the aim of increasing understanding of the context of this study.

References

Adamolekun, B., Levy, L. F., Mielke, J., & Zhande, G. (1996). The pattern of utilization of EEG services in Harare, Zimbabwe. *The Central African Journal of Medicine, 42*(11), 319–322.

Al-Adawi, S., Al-Salmy, H., Martin, R. G., Al-Naamani, A., Prabhakar, S., Deleu, D., & Dorvlo, A. S. (2003). Patient's perspective on epilepsy: Self-knowledge among Omanis. *Seizure, 12*(1), 11–18.

Assogba, K., Waklasti, P., Kombate, D., Apetse, K., & Balogou, A. A. K. (2017). *Epilepsy treatment failure associated factors in Togo.* Paper presented at the 3rd African Epilepsy Congress, Dakar Senegal, May 5–7, 2017.

Balde, E. S., Cisse, F. A., Toure, A., Kouyate, Y., & Balde, A. M. (2017). *Place of traditional medicine in management of epilepsy in Guinea.* Paper presented at the 3rd African Epilepsy Congress, Dakar Senegal, May 5–7, 2017.

Ball, D. E., Mielke, J., Adamolekun, B., Mundanda, T., & McLean, J. (2000). Community leader education to increase epilepsy attendance at clinics in Epworth, Zimbabwe. *Epilepsia, 41*(8), 1044–1045.

Ball, D. E., & Taderera, A. (2003). Development of drug use indicators for epilepsy. *The Central African Journal of Medicine, 49*(11–12), 134–138.

Birbeck, G. L. (2008). In memoriam: Jens Karl-Heinrich Mielke, MBChB, MRCP (1960–2008). *Neurology, 71*(4), 239–239.

Bishop, M. (2002). Barriers to employment among people with epilepsy: Report of a focus group. *Journal of Vocational Rehabilitation, 17*(4), 281–286.

Bradley, P. M., Lindsay, B., & Fleeman, N. (2016). Care delivery and self management strategies for adults with epilepsy. *Cochrane Database of Systematic Review, 2.* doi:10.1002/14651858.CD006244.pub3

Butau, T., & Piachaud, J. (1993). Knowledge and beliefs about epilepsy in mothers of children with epilepsy: A view from a developing country. *The Central African Journal of Medicine, 39*(9), 183–188.

Coker, M. F., Bhargava, S., Fitzgerald, M., & Doherty, C. P. (2011). What do people with epilepsy know about their condition? Evaluation of a subspecialty clinic population. *Seizure, 20*(1), 55–59. doi:10.1016/j.seizure.2010.10.007

Day, K. (2008). Quality of life: The role of psychological resilience. Thesis-Clinical Psychology Document Number 155 University of Edinburgh, Edinburgh.

Dewa, E., January, J., Nyati-Jokomo, Z., Mafaune, P. T., Muteti, S., & Maradzika, J. (2014). Non-attendance of treatment review visits among epileptic patients in a rural district, Zimbabwe. *Journal of Public Health in Africa, 5*(2), 73–76. doi:10.4081/jphia.2014.351

Doumbe, J., Bikek, D. P., Kuate, C., & Njamnsh, A. (2017). *Knowledge, attitudes and practices of healthcare professionals with respect to epilepsy in public hospitals in Douala.* Paper presented at the 3rd African Epilepsy Congress, Dakar Senegal, May 5–7, 2017.

Duggan, M. B. (2013). Epilepsy and its effects on children and families in rural Uganda. *African Health Sciences, 13*(3), 613–623. doi:10.4314/ahs.v13i3.14

Edward, K., Cook, M., & Giandinoto, J. (2015). An integrative review of the benefits of self-management interventions for adults with epilepsy. *Epilepsy & Behavior, 45*, 195–204.

Erickson, W. A., von Schrader, S., Bruyère, S. M., & VanLooy, S. A. (2014). The employment environment: Employer perspectives, policies, and practices regarding the employment of persons with disabilities. *Rehabilitation Counseling Bulletin, 57*(4), 195–208. doi:10.1177/0034355213509841

Geerts, A., Brouwer, O., van Donselaar, C., Stroink, H., Peters, B., Peeters, E., & Arts, W. F. (2011). Health perception and socioeconomic status following childhood-onset epilepsy: The Dutch study of epilepsy in childhood. *Epilepsia (Series 4), 52*(12), 2192–2202. doi:10.1111/j.1528-1167.2011.03294.x

Halima, F. S. N., Ndiaye, M., Magnerou, A. M., Hamza, H., Sow, A. D., & Ndiaye, M. M. (2017). *Lives of people with epilepsy at work in Dakar.* Paper presented at the 3rd African Epilepsy Congress, Dakar Senegal, May 5–7, 2017.

Holland, P., Lane, S., Whitehead, M., Marson, A. G., & Jacoby, A. (2009). Labor market participation following onset of seizures and early epilepsy: Findings from a UK cohort. *Epilepsia (Series 4), 50*(5), 1030–1039. doi:10.1111/j.1528-1167.2008.01819.x

Hounsossou, C. H., Queneuille, J. P., Ibinga, E., Preux, P. M., Dalmay, F., Druet-Cabanac, M., & Houinato, D. (2015). Knowledge, attitudes, and behavior among key people involved in the employment of people with epilepsy in southern Benin. *Epilepsy & Behavior, 42*, 153–158. doi:10.1016/j.yebeh.2014.10.022

International Labour Organisation (ILO). (1993). *Resolution concerning the International Classification of Status in Employment (ICSE).* Retrieved July 8, 2016 from https://www.ilo.org/global/statistics-and-databases/standards-and-guidelines/resolutions-adopted-by-international-conferences-of-labour-statisticians/WCMS_087562/lang--en/index.htm

International Labour Organisation (ILO). (2001). *Code of practice for managing disability in the workplace.* Retrieved March 12, 2016 from https://www.ilo.org/public/english/standards/relm/gb/docs/gb282/pdf/tmemdw-2.pdf

International Labour Organisation (ILO). (2005a). *Employment of people with disabilities a human rights approach.* Retrieved December 8, 2016 from https://www.ilo.org/wcmsp5/groups/public/---ed_emp/---ifp_skills/documents/publication/wcms_107853.pdf

International Labour Organisation (ILO). (2005b). *Livelihood and employment creation.* Geneva: ILO.

International Labour Organisation (ILO). (2007). *Skills development through Community Based Rehabilitation (CBR: A good practice guide).* Geneva: ILO.

International Labour Organisation (ILO). (2013). *Inclusion of people with disabilities in Zambia.* Lusaka: ILO.

International Labour Organisation (ILO). (2015). *Disability inclusion strategy and action plan 2014–17.* Retrieved October 1, 2016 from https://www.ilo.org/global/topics/disability-and-work/WCMS_475650/lang--en/index.htm

International Labour Organisation (ILO). (2016). *Decent work and the 2030 Agenda for sustainable development.* Retrieved October 13, 2016. from https://www.ilo.org/global/topics/sdg-2030/lang--en/index.htm

International Labour Organisation (ILO). (2017). *Disability and work.* Retrieved January 26, 2017 from https://ilo.org/global/topics/disability-and-work/WCMS_475650/lang--en/index.htm

Jacoby, A., & Baker, G. A. (2008). Quality-of-life trajectories in epilepsy: A review of the literature. *Epilepsy & Behavior, 12*(4), 557–571. doi:10.1016/j.yebeh.2007.11.013

Jacoby, A., Gorry, J., & Baker, G. A. (2005). Employers' attitudes to employment of people with epilepsy: Still the same old story? *Epilepsia (Series 4), 46*(12), 1978–1987. doi:10.1111/j.1528-1167.2005.00345.x

Ju, S., Roberts, E., & Zhang, D. (2013). Employer attitudes toward workers with disabilities: A review of research in the past decade. *Journal of Vocational Rehabilitation, 38*(2), 113–123.

Lim, K. S., Wo, S. W., Wong, M. H., & Tan, C. T. (2013). Impact of epilepsy on employment in Malaysia. *Epilepsy & Behavior, 27*(1), 130–134. doi:10.1016/j.yebeh.2012.12.034

Madzokere, C. (1997). Life experiences of people with epilepsy. A study of Highfield high density residential area in Harare, Zimbabwe. *EPICADEC News (Biennual Newsletter of Foundation Epilepsy Care Developing Countries), 10*(97), 19–21.

Manungo, J. (1993). Childhood epilepsy in Zimbabwe. *Tropical and Geographical Medicine, 45*(5), 246–247.

Mielke, J. (2006). Phenobarbital for convulsive epilepsy at primary care level. *Lancet Neurology, 5*(1), 17–18. doi:10.1016/S1474-4422(05)70254-4

Mielke, J., Adamolekun, B., Ball, D., & Mundanda, T. (1997). Knowledge and attitudes of teachers towards epilepsy in Zimbabwe. *Acta Neurologica Scandinavica, 96*(3), 133–137.

Mielke, J., Sebit, M., & Adamolekun, B. (2000). The impact of epilepsy on the quality of life of people with epilepsy in Zimbabwe: A pilot study. *Seizure, 9*(4), 259–264.

Morenikeji, K. Taofiki, S., Olusegun, A. Ayoade, A., Ajiboye, J., & Olaniyan, S. (2017). *Knowledge of, perceptions of and attitudes towards schoolchildren with epilepsy among teachers in south-western Nigeria.* Paper presented at the 3rd African Epilepsy Congress, Dakar Senegal, May 5–7, 2017.

Mugumbate, J., & Mushonga, J. (2013). Myths, perceptions, and incorrect knowledge surrounding epilepsy in rural Zimbabwe: A study of the villagers in Buhera District. *Epilepsy & Behavior, 27*(1), 144–147. doi:10.1016/j.yebeh.2012.12.036

Mugumbate, J., & Nyanguru, A. (2013). Measuring the challenges of people with epilepsy in Harare, Zimbabwe. *Neurology Asia, 18*(1), 29–33.

Munn, Z. (2008). Care delivery and self-management strategies for adults with epilepsy. *Journal of Advanced Nursing, 64*, 455–456.

Mushi, D., Hunter, E., Mtuya, C., Mshana, G., Aris, E. & Walker, R. (2011). Social-cultural aspects of epilepsy in Kilimanjaro Region, Tanzania: Knowledge and experience among patients and carers. *Epilepsy and Behaviour, 20*, 338–343.

Nhachi, C. F., & Mwaluko, G. M. (1990). Therapeutic drug monitoring (TDM): An aid to antiepileptic drug (AED) therapy in Zimbabwe: A review. *East African Medical Journal, 67*(5), 311–318.

Nuhu, F. T., Fawole, J. O., Babalola, O. J., Ayilara, O. O., & Sulaiman, Z. T. (2010). Social consequences of epilepsy: A study of 231 Nigerian patients. *Annals of African Medicine, 9*(3), 170–175. doi:10.4103/1596-3519.68360

Obiako, R. O., Iwuozo E. U., Kehinde, A. J., Sheikh, T. L. Ekele, N. et al. (2014). Perceptions of psychosocial impacts of epilepsy by affected persons in Northern Nigeria. *African Journal of Neurological Sciences, 13*(1), 55–63.

Quereshi, C., Standing, H. C., Swai, A., Hunter, E., Walker, R., & Owens, S. (2017). Barriers to access to education for young people with epilepsy in Northern Tanzania: A qualitative interview and focus group study involving teachers, parents and young people with epilepsy. *Epilepsy & Behavior, 72*, 145–149. doi:10.1016/j.yebeh.2017.04.005

Richardson, C. E. (2002). The metatheory of resilience and resiliency. *Journal of Clinical Psychology, 58*(3), 307–321.

Ring, A., Jacob, A., Baker, G., Marson, A., & Whitehead, M. (2016). Does the concept of resilience contribute to understanding good quality of life in the context of epilepsy? *Epilepsy & Behavior, 56*, 153–164.

Saburi, G. (2011). Stressors of caregivers of school-age children with epilepsy and use of community resources. *Neuroscience Nursing, 43*(3), 1–12. doi:10.1097/JNN. 0b013e31821456f6

Saburi, G., Mapanga, K. G., & Mapanga, M. B. (2006). Perceived family reactions and quality of life of adults with epilepsy. *Neuroscience Nursing, 38*(3), 156.

Sang-Ahm, L. (2005). What we confront with employment of people with epilepsy in Korea. *Epilepsia, 46*(Suppl 1), 57–58.

Sebit, M. B., & Mielke, J. (2005). Epilepsy in Sub-Saharan Africa: Its socio-demography, aetiology, diagnosis and EEG characteristics in Harare, Zimbabwe. *East African Medical Journal, 82*(3), 128–137.

Sillanpää, M., & Schmidt, D. (2010). Long-term employment of adults with childhood-onset epilepsy: A prospective population-based study. *Epilepsia (Series 4), 51*(6), 1053–1060. doi:10.1111/j.1528-1167.2009.02505.x

Smeets, V., van Lierop, B., Vanhoutvin, J., Aldenkamp, A., & Nijhuis, F. (2007). Epilepsy and employment: Literature review. *Epilepsy & Behaviour, 10*, 354–362.

Soumaila, B., Adji, D. B., Maiga, Y., Hrouna, M., Touré, K., Ndiaye, M., & Adéhossi, E. (2017). *Epilepsy in schools of a rural community in Niger: A teacher-based survey.* Paper presented at the 3rd African Epilepsy Congress, Dakar Senegal, May 5-7, 2017.

Sung, C., Muller, V., Jones, J. E., & Fong, C. (2014). Vocational rehabilitation service patterns and employment outcomes of people with epilepsy. *Epilepsy Research, 108*(8), 1469–1479. doi:10.1016/j.eplepsyres.2014.06.016

Taylor, J., Jacob, A., Baker, G., Marson, A., Ring, A., & Whitehead, M. (2011). Factors predictive of resilience and vulnerability in new-onset epilepsy. *Epilepsia, 52*(3), 610–618.

United Nations (UN). (2015). *Sustainable development goals: 17 Goals to transform the world.* Retrieved November 12, 2015 from https://www.un.org/sustainabledevelopment/ economic-growth/

Vyas, M. V., Wong, A., Yang, J. M., Thistle, P., & Lee, L. (2016). The spectrum of neurological presentations in an outpatient clinic of rural Zimbabwe. *Journal of the Neurological Sciences, 362*, 263–265. doi:10.1016/j.jns.2016.01.065

Winkler, A. S., Mayer, M., Ombay, M., Mathias, B., Schmutzhard, E., & Jilek-Aall, L. (2009). Attitudes towards African traditional medicine and Christian spiritual healing regarding treatment of epilepsy in a rural community of northern Tanzania. *African Journal Traditional Complementary Alternative Medicine, 7*(2), 162–170.

Wo, M. C. M., Lim, K. S., Choo, W. Y., & Tan, C. T. (2015). Employability in people with epilepsy: A systematic review. *Epilepsy Research, 116*, 67–78. doi:10.1016/j. eplepsyres.2015.06.016

8 Initiatives on epilepsy in the Global South

In the Global South, various initiatives have been implemented to improve the quality of life of people with epilepsy and their families. This chapter provides an overview of epilepsy in Africa, Latin America, the Caribbean, Asia and the Pacific and the Middle East and North Africa (MENA). It will describe important programmes and achievements in each region, as well as the challenges they face, such as healthcare access, cultural attitudes and resource availability. This chapter will highlight the work of organisations and associations in these areas, explaining their roles and impact. Key features and difficulties specific to each region will be discussed, showing how these factors influence the management and understanding of epilepsy. At the end of this chapter, the main themes and common issues across all regions will be summarised, providing a broader view of global trends, challenges and successful approaches in dealing with epilepsy.

Epilepsy in Africa

This section discusses epilepsy in the continent of Africa, focusing on sub-Sahara Africa which falls under the World Health Organisation (WHO) Africa Regional Office. Before the 1990s, there were very few activities on epilepsy in the African region. More resourced countries like South Africa had activities, but they were limited to the country or connected to countries of Europe because of colonisation. In 1997, the GCAE was initiated. In 2000, the African declaration of epilepsy was made in Dakar, Senegal. A few years later, Zimbabwe took part as a demonstration project site until 2005. In 2007, Epilepsy Support Association of Uganda hosted an African regional meeting in Kampala. A few years later, Zambia Epilepsy hosted a regional meeting in Lusaka. In 2012, the first Regional Epilepsy Congress was held in Lusaka, Zambia, and the second one was held in 2014 in Cape Town, South Africa. Subsequent Congress were held in Dakar, Senegal in 2017 and Kampala, Uganda in 2019. A key development in 2019 was the founding of the Epilepsy Alliance Africa which focuses on the whole of Africa (North and South) and is for both lay people and professionals.

The African Declaration on Epilepsy, titled Epilepsy: A healthcare priority in Africa was agreed at a meeting held in Dakar, Senegal, Africa on 5 and 6 May 2000. African governments were asked to create national plans to address important

DOI: 10.4324/9781003602866-8

areas. This included ensuring access to trained staff, modern diagnostic tools, antiepileptic medication and surgical treatments, as well as promoting information sharing, prevention and social inclusion. Governments were also asked to educate and train healthcare workers about epilepsy and raise awareness among those affected and the general public that it is a treatable neurological condition. Efforts were needed to stop discrimination, especially in schools and workplaces. Additionally, the prevention and treatment of epilepsy were to be included in national health plans for related issues like maternal and child health, mental health, infections, head injuries and other health programmes. Governments were encouraged to involve the public and private sectors, as well as NGOs, in local activities for the Global Campaign against Epilepsy, promote cooperation with traditional health systems, and support research on epilepsy. Declaring a National Epilepsy Day and encouraging regional and continental cooperation were also important steps in tackling this issue.

Information box 8.1 The Zimbabwe epilepsy model

In Zimbabwe, the management of epilepsy falls under the Mental Health Unit in the Ministry of Health and Child Welfare. Medical and healthcare practice is regulated by the Essential Medicines List and Standard Treatment Guidelines for Zimbabwe, commonly referred to as the Essential Drugs List for Zimbabwe (EDLIZ) (Government of Zimbabwe, 2011). The guidelines authorise health workers, mostly medical/psychiatric practitioners and nurses, to diagnose and treat epilepsy and provide training standards for them. The Ministry of Health and Child Care follows a public health approach (WHO, 1978) with services delivered at three levels:

1　Primary healthcare is the first level of contact individuals, families and communities have with the healthcare system.
2　Secondary healthcare is offered by a specialist practitioner or medical facility upon referral by a primary—community-based—care provider.
3　Tertiary healthcare is provided by specialists working in a centre that has dedicated personnel and facilities for special investigation and treatment, usually on referral from primary or secondary medical care personnel.

Primary healthcare facilities are usually within walking distance of most communities, that is, 10 kilometres or more (Choruma, 2006). Sebit and Mielke (2005) reported that the five major referral hospitals, all of which are in urban areas, offered limited services for people with epilepsy, while private health facilities in urban areas were beyond the reach of most Zimbabweans. There was a shortage of antiepileptic medicines and, often, people with epilepsy could not afford the cost of travel, medicines, tests and hospital fees. Mielke, Sebit and Adamolekun (2000) reported increasing concern that 'patient-related concerns were not being addressed. These include important social and psychological issues, such as advice for employers and employees, advocacy at the work-place and daily functioning issues for more severely disabled PWE' (p. 260).

The ESF and the ERCZ are the main non-government organisations dedicated to supporting people with epilepsy in Zimbabwe—attempted to address these issues. The ESF has a social rehabilitation unit and a clinic with an EEG. The ESF treatment of epilepsy also provides advocacy services and administrative support for income-generating projects, and works to influence policy change (Epilepsy Support Foundation [ESF], 2012). Its rehabilitation centre offers health education, disagnosis, treatment, dispensary counselling and limited psychosocial and economic interventions. Health education programmes include awareness-raising events during National Epilepsy Awareness Week, International Epilepsy Day and Purple Day. ESF also runs support groups in some areas of the country and its personnel included people with epilepsy. The Zimbabwe League Against Epilepsy (ZLAE) is the only other NGO 'promoting epilepsy awareness, treatment and providing back up support to people with epilepsy' (Mugumbate & Nyanguru, 2013, p. 29).

There is no dedicated plan, programme or law for epilepsy in Zimbabwe.

Epilepsy in Latin America

The Pan American Health Organisation (PAHO) is the WHO Regional Office in this region, which includes the Caribbean region. PAHO has a Strategy and Plan of Action on Epilepsy 2012–2021 that was put in place in 2011 to support programmes and legislation; health and treatment, education and sensitisation and information systems strengthening. By 2016, progress had been made. For example, out of a target of 25, 18 countries had national epilepsy programmes in place and 10 had developed epilepsy legislation (PAHO, 2018). However, death as a result of epilepsy was still very high (0.84 per 100,000 people) but being as high 1.04 per 100,000 in some countries against a target of 0.8 per 100,000 (PAHO, 2018). A timeline of epilepsy-focused activities in the region is as follows:

- 2000 – Latin American Epilepsy Congress started.
- 2000 – Declaration of Santiago on Epilepsy in Latin America.
- 2011 – PAHO's 51st Directing Council approved its Strategy and Plan of Action on Epilepsy 2012–2021.
- 2015 – PAHO conducted a mid-term evaluation of the Regional Plan's indicators.
- 0000 – Latin American Epilepsy Day, 9 September.
- 2013 – Report on Epilepsy in Latin America and the Caribbean (LAC).
- 2007 – Latin American Academy of Epilepsy (LAAE).
- 2003 – Epilepsy demonstration project in the regions of Campinas and São Jose do Rio Preto, in the Sao Paulo State, Brazil as part of the GCAE (Li & Sander, 2003).

> **Information box 8.2   The burden of epilepsy going down in Latin America**
>
> Pacheco-Barrios et al. (2021, online) analysed data on Latin America and Caribbean and concluded that
>
>> Over the past 30 years, the epilepsy burden in LAC has decreased; however, it is still high and contributes significantly to the global epilepsy burden. This burden is YLD predominant, mostly in the youth and elderly. However, mortality and premature death are still higher than in other GBD regions, particularly in male older adults. Alcohol use is the only available risk factor, and the SDI is an essential regional determinant for burden and mortality (higher SDI, less burden). The high mortality and YLLs in the region, mainly in the elderly, suggest a lack of access to adequate pharmacological treatment. Therefore, there is an urgent need for planning in LAC. This should include prompt access to treatment in all levels of care, underscoring the strengthening of primary care and the systematic reduction of stigma and marginalization of people with epilepsy in LAC.
>
> This research by Pacheco-Barrios et al. (2021) could be more relevant to Latin America but maybe not so for the Caribbean Islands.

Epilepsy in the Caribbean Islands

This region is made up of countries like Antigua and Barbuda, Barbados, Dominica, Grenada, Jamaica, St Kitts and Nevis, St Lucia, Trinidad and Tobago and Jamaica. The key organisations for epilepsy include the PAHO which also covers Latin America and the Epilepsy Society of the Caribbean (ESC). An important programme of action for epilepsy in this region is the PAHO Epilepsy Plan of Action. The North American Regional Caribbean Congress on Epilepsy is an important meeting. In this region, more than 50% of the population does not receive epilepsy treatment owing to poverty, stigma and exclusion (PAHO, 2018). In 2015, for example, Epilepsy Foundation of Guyana reported that the country had no practicing neurologist, no electroencephalogram (EEG) and very few older AEDs types with limited access (PAHO, 2018). However, Barbados reported a 23.7% decrease in mortality in 20 years due to the availability of facilities and practitioners which made be possible for epilepsy to be viewed as a medically treatable condition (PAHO, 2018). However, the cost of treatment was high especially considering that people with epilepsy require long term care. Jamaican Epilepsy Association (JEA) reported similar challenges but mainly limited personnel. In Grenada, the major challenge reported was social attitudes that do not support medical treatment although the state has services for epilepsy at the primary, secondary and tertiary levels. Lack of research was another challenge reported. St Lucia reported a system with a bit more health facilities for epilepsy although for some services patients had to go to Martinique, another country. The situation reported in Trinidad and Tobago was more positive—eight neurologists, eight neurosurgeons, a neuropsychologist, one paediatric neurologist, social workers and neurophysiology technicians (PAHO, 2018).

Epilepsy in Asia and the Pacific

This region is vast. It consists of the World Health Organization Regional Office for South-East Asia (SEARO) with about 2 billion people in 11 countries and the Western Pacific Region with about 1.9 billion people in 37 countries. There are differences in the size, cultures and resource levels of each country. China and India, for example, have huge populations while Maldives is very small. Countries like Aotearoa (New Zealand), Australia, China, Singapore, Japan and South Korea are rich, but Papua New Guinea, Indonesia and Cambodia are not. Nauru, Macao (China) and Singapore are 100% urban, yet Viet Nam, Vanuatu, Samoa, Cambodia and are below 25%. The richer countries have key resources for epilepsy, which are policies, specialists, trained primary healthcare workers, epilepsy associations and epilepsy equipment while the poorer countries like Palau and Nauru have no specialists and other important resources.

In the Pacific region, the percentage of people with epilepsy who are not on treatment can be as high as 95% (WHO, 2000). Further, the awareness gap can be just as high. To reduce these gaps, the Asian and Oceanian declaration on epilepsy was agreed at an Asian and Oceanian Epilepsy Organization (AOEO) summit held in New Delhi, India in 2000 (WHO, 2000). Further, in 2001, the Regional Strategy for Mental Health was endorsed by the 52nd Regional Committee of the Western Pacific Region in Brunei Darussalam. The strategy adopted epilepsy as a priority. As part of the GCAE, China was selected to host a demonstration project under the GCAE.

Information box 8.3   Key challenges in the Pacific region

The WHO (2000, p. 10) reports that the key challenges in this region were:

- There are no or insufficient epidemiological data, resulting in unreliable estimates of the burden of epilepsy in most countries of the Western Pacific Region.
- Little attention is given to public education on epilepsy, so that misunderstanding and social stigma persists largely unchallenged.
- Neurologists and health services for epilepsy are lacking or not properly distributed.
- Most people with epilepsy are not diagnosed and treated appropriately.

- Proper legislation on and coordination of epilepsy among government sectors (such as public health, education and labour) are needed.
- Superstition and unscientific and popular therapies need to be combated or tested using scientific methods. Fraudulent therapies need to be controlled by law.
- Further research on epilepsy, especially on the public health aspects, is needed.
- Professional and lay organisations, epilepsy foundations and networks of epilepsy centres need to be developed.

The Epilepsy Management at a Primary Health Level demonstration project in Central China was completed in 2005 and included an epidemiological survey, an intervention study and an educational programme in the provinces Heilongjiang, Ningxia, Henan, Shanxi and Jiangsu. The provinces had a total population of over 2.5 million people at the time. The survey showed that prevalence was higher than estimated (7 per 1,000 or 0.7%), active epilepsy prevalence of 4.6 per 1,000 (0.46%) and treatment gap was about 7%. Compliance with treatment was very high, 95%. The intervention included mandatory training for primary healthcare physicians on diagnosis, treatment and compliance, supervised by local neurologists.

The noun epilepsy is derived from the Greek word *epilambanein* and means to be seized (Shorvon, 2024). Both the nouns epilepsy and seizures misrepresent the condition and can result in stigma (Kim, Kang, Lee, Huh, & Lee, 2014). Some countries in Asia have changed the name epilepsy and seizure because these names promote stigma (Li, 2014). In Korea, the word for epilepsy is expressed as gan-jil, 간질,癎疾 and comes from dian-xian 癲癎 which refers to craziness or madness. The Korean Epilepsy Association and Korean Medical Association changed this name in 2010/2011 to noi-jeon-jeung 뇌전증 or 'cerebro-electric disorder' (Li, 2014). Later, Hong Kong, China and Japan changed from epilepsy. The debate to change in other countries is ongoing (Kim et al., 2014).

Epilepsy in the MENA

Epilepsy understanding in the MENA, which has 22 countries is largely shaped by tradition and religion (Kissani et al., 2020; Al-Khateeb & Al-Khateeb, 2014). This region is also known as the Arab or Muslim region because of its majority Muslim population. The WHO Eastern Mediterranean Regional Office is the largest health organisation. In 2003, in Cairo, Egypt, the MENA region agreed and launched a Declaration on Epilepsy as part of the GCAE. They advocated for more government involvement in funding and managing epilepsy (Khan, 2015). This call was also extended to the private sector and non-government organisations. The declaration was guided by several considerations, which are still relevant in the MENA region today. In the region, epilepsy is often not understood as a treatable condition, and there is limited knowledge that most people with the condition can lead productive lives with relatively cheap and effective treatment. In many parts of the Eastern Mediterranean region, especially in rural areas, people have no access to proper healthcare or treatment. Information about epilepsy, trained experts, diagnostic facilities, antiepileptic drugs and surgery are often not available or affordable due to geographic, financial, cultural, or communication barriers. Epilepsy has serious physical, psychological and social effects on those affected and their families, with the impact being especially severe in children and teenagers. Moreover, epilepsy does not receive enough attention in national health plans in many countries in the region.

Crosscutting themes from the regions

A major theme is that the treatment gap is very high in all regions of the Global South, meaning the physical, social and economic burden of epilepsy remains very high. The physical burden is evident in the large number of individuals living with uncontrolled seizures, significant mortality rates and increased disability. Socially, people with epilepsy face stigma, exclusion and injustice, which further complicate their lives. Economically, the challenges include widespread poverty, the high cost of treatment and the loss of income and employment opportunities. This chapter highlights these severe burdens and underscores the urgent need for more effective strategies and support systems to address them. Despite various regional efforts and achievements, the ongoing challenges reveal the critical need for comprehensive and targeted approaches to reduce the treatment gap and improve the quality of life for those affected by epilepsy in resource-limited settings. The IGAP programme, which started in 2022 and runs through 2031, will be a valuable global policy measure in addressing these challenges. By providing a structured framework for action, IGAP aims to enhance epilepsy care and support across worldwide. The next chapter deals with global actions on epilepsy, including the IGAP programme.

References

African Declaration on Epilepsy. (2000). *Epilepsy: A healthcare priority in Africa*. Dakar: African Commission on Epilepsy.

Al-Khateeb, J. M., & Al-Khateeb, A. J. (2014). Research on psychosocial aspects of epilepsy in Arab countries: A review of literature. *Epilepsy & Behavior, 31*, 256–262. doi:10.1016/j.yebeh.2013.09.033

Choruma, T. (2006). *The forgotten tribe: People with disabilities in Zimbabwe*. London: Progressio.

Epilepsy Support Foundation (ESF). (2012). *Annual report*. Harare: ESF.

Government of Zimbabwe. (2011). *Essential Drug List of Zimbabwe (EDLIZ)*. Harare: Ministry of Health and Child Care Zimbabwe.

Khan, S. A. (2015). Epilepsy awareness in Saudi Arabia. *Neurosciences (Riyadh, Saudi Arabia), 20*(3), 205–206. doi:10.17712/nsj.2015.3.20150338

Kim, H. D., Kang, H., Lee, S. A., Huh, K., & Lee, B. (2014). Changing name of epilepsy in Korea; cerebroelectric disorder (noi-jeon-jeung, 뇌전증,腦電症). *Epilepsia, 55*(3), 384–386. doi:10.1111/epi.12516

Kissani, N., Balili, K., Mesraoua, B., Abdulla, F., Bashar, G., Al-Baradie, R., Elsahli, R., Ibrahim, E., Al-Asmi, A., Mounir, N., Kishk, N. A., Harharah, A., Abu Aliqa, A., Honein, A., Arabi, M., & Asadi-Pooya, A. A. (2020). Epilepsy and school in the Middle East and North Africa (MENA) region: The current situation, challenges, and solutions. *Epilepsy & Behavior, 112,* 107325–107325. doi:10.1016/j.yebeh.2020.107325

Li, L. M., & Sander, J. W. A. S. (2003). National demonstration project on epilepsy in Brazil. *Arquivos de neuro-psiquiatria, 61*(1), 153–156. doi:10.1590/S0004-282X2003000100033

Li, S. (2014). Comments in response the changing name of "epilepsy" in Korea. *Epilepsia, 55*(3), *387–387.* doi:10.1111/epi.12543

Mielke, J., Sebit, M., & Adamolekun, B. (2000). The impact of epilepsy on the quality of life of people with epilepsy in Zimbabwe: A pilot study. *Seizure, 9*(4), 259–264.

Mugumbate, J., & Nyanguru, A. (2013). Measuring the challenges of people with epilepsy in Harare, Zimbabwe. *Neurology Asia, 18*(1), 29–33.

Pacheco-Barrios, K., Navarro-Flores, A., Cardenas-Rojas, A., de Melo, P. S., Uygur-Kucukseymen, E., Alva-Diaz, C., Fregni, F., & Burneo, J. G. (2021). Burden of epilepsy in Latin America and The Caribbean: A trend analysis of the Global Burden of Disease Study 1990–2019. *Lancet Regional Health. Americas, 8,* 100140. https://doi.org/10.1016/j.lana.2021.100140

Pan American Health Organization. (2018). Improving the management of epilepsy and its Comorbidities in the Caribbean. Regional Workshop (Trinidad and Tobago, 28 February–1 March 2018). Document Number: PAHO/NMH/18-028.

Sebit, M. B., & Mielke, J. (2005). Epilepsy in Sub-Saharan Africa: Its socio-demography, aetiology, diagnosis and EEG characteristics in Harare, Zimbabwe. *East African Medical Journal, 82*(3), 128–137.

Shorvon, S. (2024). Should we use the word 'epilepsy'? *Epilepsy & Behavior, 157,* 109865-. doi:10.1016/j.yebeh.2024.109865

World Health Organisation (WHO). (1978). *Declaration of Alma Ata.* International conference on PHC, Alma-Ata, USSR, 6–12 September.

World Health Organization (WHO). (2000). *Asian and Oceanian declaration on epilepsy.* New Delhi: WHO.

World Health Organization (WHO). (2003). *Eastern mediterranean declaration on epilepsy.* Retrieved from https://www.ilae.org/files/dmfile/EasternMedDeclarationEpilepsy.pdf

9 Global initiatives on epilepsy

This chapter covers global organisations, programmes and policies on epilepsy. It will begin with a summary of key global organisations and then a discussion of what constitutes policy and the importance of policies. This will lead to a discussion of previous global policies on epilepsy and how they were implemented, together with the roles of the organisations involved. The discussion will then move onto current global programmes on epilepsy focusing on the Intersectoral Global Action Plan on Epilepsy (2022–2031), its aims, goals, strategies and the organisations involved. A key discussion will be on the role of governments but also communities. This chapter will end with a discussion of policy gaps, and how these could be addressed.

Overview

Epilepsy is a condition that is prevalent throughout the world, and is found in all populations of the world. Managing the condition requires an international approach to support the work that happens at community, country, regional and continental levels. To ensure global activities are sustained and better coordinated, international organisations have been formed, and global programmes and policies have been in place, as shown in Information box 9.1.

Information box 9.1   Global organisations, policies and programmes

Global organisations	*Global policy*	*Global programmes, plans and actions*
International League Against Epilepsy (ILAE)	WHO Declaration on the: Global burden of epilepsy and the need for coordinated action at the country level to address its health, social and public knowledge implications, 2015	Global Campaign Against Epilepsy, 1997
World Health Organisation (WHO)		WHO Mental Health Gap Action Programme (mGAP), 2008
		International Epilepsy Day, since 2015
		Intersectoral global action plan on epilepsy and other neurological disorders, 2021
International Bureau for Epilepsy (IBE)		International epilepsy congresses (main one run by the ILAE and IBE)
World Federation of Neurology (WFN)		Demonstration or pilot projects
		WHO Comprehensive Mental Health Action Plan 2013–2030

DOI: 10.4324/9781003602866-9

In Information box 9.1, organisations leading epilepsy work globally were formed in Western countries. It follows then that programmes, policies and publications are Western oriented.

Global organisations

International League Against Epilepsy

The ILAE is the oldest global organisation on epilepsy. It was formed in Budapest, Hungary, Europe in 1909. Their main goals are to be the top resource for health professionals on the latest epilepsy practices, help health professionals improve their skills, promote epilepsy as a major health issue, and support research and new ideas about epilepsy.

World Health Organisation

Formed in Geneva, Switzerland, Europe in 1948, the WHO is responsible for global health and it has over the years developed programmes on mental health, neurological health, disability, primary healthcare and epilepsy. The main goals of the WHO are to make sure everyone has access to good healthcare, fight diseases and health problems, make health systems better, and help people learn how to stay healthy.

International Bureau for Epilepsy

This organisation was formed by the ILAE in Rome in 1961 (Kaculini et al., 2021) to address the social issues of epilepsy. Their main goals are to raise awareness about epilepsy, support people with epilepsy and their families, help improve services and treatments, and promote research to find better ways to manage epilepsy. They work to make sure people with epilepsy get the help and understanding they need.

World Federation of Neurology (WFN)

The WFN was formed in Brussels, Belgium, Europe in 1957 to promote neurology and brain health. It has four regions—Africa, Americas, Asia and Europe. The main goals of the WFN are to support doctors who treat brain and nervous system problems, help with training and education for medical professionals, raise awareness about brain health issues and encourage research to find better treatments and solutions.

Global programmes

Global campaign against epilepsy

Code named Out of the Shadows, the global campaign against epilepsy (GCAE) was led by the WHO, the ILAE and the IBE from 1997 to 2007 (WHO, 2007,

2004). The campaign sought to bring epilepsy 'out of the shadows' through dissemination of information about the condition and strengthening of public and private collaborations to improve epilepsy management and lessen its burden. According to the ILAE, IBE and WHO (1997), the specific mission of the campaign was to 'improve the acceptability, treatment, services and prevention of epilepsy worldwide.' However, the campaign focused more on resource-poor settings. For example, as part of the GCAE, demonstration projects that included baseline data collection, training intervention and evaluation data collection were done in China, Brazil, Senegal and Zimbabwe. According to WHO, the overall result from the four projects was that 'there are simple, cost-effective ways to treat epilepsy in low-resource settings'. Another important aspect of the GCAE were the declarations. There were also regional reports and conferences. With this campaign, different regions of the world agreed on declarations that we launched and became a rallying point. The declarations included the African Declaration on epilepsy agreed in Dakar, Senegal, in 2000. Other declarations included the European Declaration (Heidelberg, Germany) (1998), Declaration of Santiago on Epilepsy in Latin America Santiago (Chile) (2000), Asian-Oceanian Declaration on Epilepsy (New Delhi, India) (2000), the North American Declaration on Epilepsy (Los Angeles, U.S.A.) (2000) and the Eastern Mediterranean Declaration on Epilepsy (Cairo, Egypt) (2003). The key themes of the declarations were:

- Public education
- Community-based control and prevention programmes
- Legislative reform
- Investment in research
- Lay and professional epilepsy organisations
- Information exchange and inter-country cooperation

The GCAE improved prioritisation of epilepsy in many parts of the globe, and activities were recorded in over 100 countries (ILAE, 2008). Some of the benefits were:

1 Many countries carried out projects to reduce the treatment gap and death because of epilepsy.
2 There was increased training and education of health professionals.
3 Epilepsy was integrated into primary, secondary and tertiary healthcare systems.
4 Laws and policies were improved.

However, a key challenge was that activities did not go up as expected. In response, in 2009, a global taskforce was formed to spearhead activities and to find synergies with other activities that were happening outside the GCAE. In 2019, the taskforce became the Global Outreach, with a responsibility to increase cooperation in epilepsy education and service delivery globally.

Mental health gap action programme (mGAP)

The mhGAP is another global programme initiated by the WHO in 2007 to scale up care for mental, neurological and substance use disorders (WHO, 2008). The focus was prevention and management of selected mental health conditions in low-to middle-income countries. The selected conditions were depression, schizophrenia, suicide, epilepsy, dementia, alcohol and drug use disorders and child mental health. The mhGAP package consists of interventions for prevention and management for each of these priority conditions. For epilepsy, this programme involved demonstration projects in Ghana, Mozambique, Myanmar and Viet Nam.

International epilepsy days

The key to successful management of epilepsy is correct knowledge about the condition. This is mainly achieved through public awareness. Awareness for epilepsy has taken a global dimension, mainly with the starting of International Epilepsy Day in 2015. The day is supported by the International Bureau for Epilepsy and the International League Against Epilepsy. Other international epilepsy days of significance include International Epilepsy Caring Day celebrated on 28 June and was started in 2007 by China Association Against Epilepsy Bureau for Epilepsy and the Purple Day started in Canada in 2008 and is celebrated on 26 March (Mugumbate et al., 2023).

Demonstration and pilot projects

Demonstration and pilot projects serve a purpose of testing interventions and producing prototypes that could be scaled up in the same country or globally. Several such projects have been implemented in the Global South. Eight projects carried out in China, Brazil, Senegal, Zimbabwe (2002–2005), Mozambique (2013–2017), Ghana (2012), Myanmar and Vietnam will be summarised focusing on aims, objectives, methods, results, implications and impact.

GCAE pilot projects

GCAE projects consisted of project teams that worked with local medical and social associations to survey the prevalence of epilepsy and test the feasibility of training non-specialist health workers to manage epilepsy at the primary care level (Wolf, 2002).

Information box 9.2   Global campaign against epilepsy pilot projects

Country details	Aim, objectives and methods	Results, implications and impact
China Heilongjiang, Ningxia, Henan, Shanxi, Jiangsu and Shanghai provinces	Aim: To generate procedures that would improve the identification and management of people with convulsive forms of epilepsy, in rural and semi-rural areas of the country, within the existing primary healthcare system and with community participation, to develop a model of epilepsy treatment at primary health level that could be applied nationwide. Main objectives: To assess current management practices (identification, treatment and follow-up) of patients with convulsive forms of epilepsy in rural and semi-rural areas of the country; to estimate: (a) the prevalence of active forms of convulsive epilepsy, (b) the scale of the treatment gap via an active case finding methodology and (c) changes the project may bring to these figures in the study area; to ascertain the knowledge, attitudes and practice of epilepsy among health practitioners at primary health level prior to the study and after they have undergone training for epilepsy; to develop technical norms for the identification, education, treatment and follow-up of patients with epilepsy at primary healthcare level; to carry out a feasibility study, by primary healthcare doctors, of the treatment of convulsive forms of epilepsy using phenobarbital; to promote public awareness about epilepsy via an educational programme aimed at the community and to develop local advocacy and support groups for people with epilepsy.	Results showed a minimum lifetime prevalence rate of 6.2/1,000 and a prevalence of active epilepsy of 4.5/1,000. Results show that if physicians are provided with basic training to manage epilepsy, they could do so successfully and in a cost-effective way using phenobarbital. The treatment gap reduced by about 13% because of physician training and availability of cost-effective anti-epilepsy medicines between 2001 and 2004. A major implication of this study was that phenobarbital treatment as a first option for epilepsy was extended in China and by 2007, the treatment project has been replicated in 12 provinces (Wang et al., 2008; Yang et al., 2012).

Country details	Aim, objectives and methods	Results, implications and impact
	Methodology: This demonstration project was composed of three parts: an epidemiological estimation to provide a realistic estimation of the prevalence of untreated active epilepsy in the study areas; service delivery (intervention study) to cover the issues of diagnosis, phenobarbital treatment, follow-up referral networks; and educational, social and community intervention to cover the educational and social aspects of the project.	
Brazil District of Baro Geraldo in Campinas; and Districts of Santo Antonio and Jaguar in So Jos do Rio Preto	Aim: Testing the feasibility of diagnosing and treating epilepsy at primary care level with rational use of the first-line antiepileptic drugs (phenobarbital, phenytoin, carbamazepine and valproic acid) in order to integrate epilepsy management into the existing primary health delivery system in a sustainable manner. Main objectives: To generate procedures that will improve the identification and management of people with epilepsy in urban areas within the existing primary healthcare system and with community participation; and to develop a model of epilepsy treatment at primary health level that can be applied nationwide. Methodology: Epidemiological estimation; service delivery (intervention study); and education, social and community intervention.	As a result, the approach used in the project was recommended for implementation nationwide (Min & Sander, 2003; Li, Fernandes, de Boer, Prilipko, & Sander, 2007).
Senegal Pikine Health District in Dakar with a population of 480,000 living in villages, resettlement houses and squatters homes	Aim: to decrease the treatment gap and to develop a model of epilepsy care in terms of identification, treatment, prevention, education, training and research.	The Demonstration Project in Pikine revealed that the public health methodology applied was effective, despite the difficulties related to the context, and could be extended to the rest of Senegal (Mugumbate, 2010).

Country details	Aim, objectives and methods	Results, implications and impact
	Main objectives: To evaluate knowledge, attitude and practice about epilepsy; to assess local cultural beliefs and health-seeking strategies; to develop epilepsy training modules; to strengthen health personnel's capacity to detect and manage epilepsy; to ameliorate access to and availability of antiepileptic drugs; to improve the prevention of epilepsy; to promote general awareness about epilepsy and to fight the stigma surrounding the condition, to set up local support groups; and to reduce the social, economic and professional burden faced by people with epilepsy. Methodology: Epidemiological survey, training of health professionals and teachers and public educational interventions (leaflets, documentary, musical and celebrity advertising) and a second survey to evaluate impacts on awareness, treatment gap, knowledge and services. Another method was setting up a drug bank for phenobarbital.	The Senegalese model was promoted in other countries, taking into account local specificity.
Zimbabwe Hwedza District with a population that time of about 90,000 people consisting of rural, farming and small urban population	Aim: to demonstrate that it is possible to improve the quality of life of people with epilepsy in rural Zimbabwe. Objectives: Establishing the prevalence of epilepsy and its treatment gap in a rural area; discerning the influence of epilepsy on the quality of life of people with epilepsy in such an area; positively influencing the physical quality of life of these people with epilepsy through a pharmaco-economic intervention (ensuring availability and accessibly of medical care and medications); and positively influencing the social quality of life of these people with epilepsy through a psychosocial intervention (a health education campaign for health staff, patients and their families and the public).	A rural community prevalence for epilepsy of 13.3/1,000 was found (Mugumbate, 2010). A treatment gap of 93% was established. Training primary healthcare workers to diagnose epilepsy (generalised convulsive seizures) was found to be effective and safe.

Country details	Aim, objectives and methods	Results, implications and impact
	Methodology: Epidemiological survey; intervention to improve treatment (training primary healthcare workers to diagnose epilepsy) and education and quality-of-life study.	Recommendations were made to the National Drug and Therapeutic Committee as well as the Ministry of Health and Child Welfare to adopt a national policy of primary healthcare worker training to diagnose and treat forms of epilepsy. Training and awareness increase attendance for treatment. The quality-of-life study showed that people are often promised that medical treatment works and was available, but this was in reality not true—at the end most people with epilepsy, their families and the community and even health workers lost confidence in medical treatments and default rates increase. Without access to affordable, accessible and available treatments, quality of life is not improved.

mhGAP pilot projects

mhGAp projects consisted of teams that collaborated with the WHO and ministries of health to promote early detection and using a community-based model of care that reached people where they lived (WHO, 2002). The overall intention was to generate a model that other low-resource settings could adopt.

Information box 9.3   mhGAP pilot projects

Country details	*Aims, objectives and methods*	*Results and implications*
Ghana Five regions comprised of 10 districts and 55 hospitals and clinics.	Aim: To expand the skills of non-specialist healthcare providers to diagnose, treat and follow up with people with epilepsy using a community-based model of care that can be replicated nationwide and in other low-resource settings. Objectives: To improve the identification and management of people with epilepsy in the existing primary healthcare system; delivering epilepsy care; training primary healthcare workers and community volunteers; raising awareness and educating communities; engaging Indigenous African, Christian and Islamic healers; and strengthening monitoring and evaluation within routine reporting systems.	The pilot project in Ghana helped increase coverage for epilepsy from 15% to 38% in four years. The project was successful in increasing coverage from 15% to 38% in the implementing districts and more than 2,700 people received treatment for the first time.
Myanmar	Aim: To expand the skills of non-specialist healthcare providers to diagnose, treat and follow up with people with epilepsy.	In Myanmar, well over 2000 healthcare providers were trained in assessment, diagnosis and treatment for people living with epilepsy. The pilot model was scaled up to reach all townships in five states/regions across the country.
Vietnam	Aim: To expand the skills of non-specialist healthcare providers to diagnose, treat and follow up with people with epilepsy.	The initiative reduced the treatment gap by 38% in project sites (Singh, Singh, Ding, Maulik, & Sander, 2023).

Country details	Aims, objectives and methods	Results and implications
Mozambique Fifty-six health facilities from 16 districts were selected from a pool of 201 units of 5 provinces—Niassa, Nampula, Zambézia, Sofala and Gaz. The population covered was 1.9 million.	Aim: To expand the skills of non-specialist healthcare providers to diagnose, treat and follow up with people with epilepsy. The first step for implementation was advocacy from the Government level to relevant stakeholders in the community. mhGAP training materials were translated and adapted to the local context. Non-specialist health providers and community health workers were trained and supervised regularly. More than 5,000 community awareness sessions were held to reduce the stigma faced by people living with epilepsy and to raise awareness of primary healthcare services available for affordable epilepsy treatment. Awareness reached more than 14,000 people per year using all 177 health professionals and 1,161 community health workers were trained and ensured services delivery for people living with epilepsy (PwE).	Treatment gap was reduced from 99% to 96%. Results were used as evidence for the Ministry of Health (MoH) to increase the purchase of antiepileptic drugs and improve delivery at the district level (Dos Santos et al., 2019).

The results from these eight pilot projects have been useful in changing policies, and in generating lessons for other countries in the Global South. However, a key issue is that demonstrations continue happening, yet the results tend to be the same, that awareness increases health seeking for epilepsy and reduces the treatment gap. Wouldn't it therefore be time for more advocacy for policy improvement and treatment, instead of generating more similar evidence? More demonstration projects have been planned as part of the intersectoral global action plan (IGAP) on epilepsy and other neurological disorders, which does seem to be a waste of resources. The pilot projects are often driven by donor money yet the donors have their own priorities of funding short-term projects in smaller areas which they are able to control.

Global policies

In 2015, the WHO adopted the Declaration on the: Global burden of epilepsy and the need for coordinated action at the country level to address its health, social and public knowledge implications (WHO, 2015). This is the current global policy on epilepsy. This policy has led to the creation of the Intersectoral Global Action Plan on Epilepsy and other Neurological Disorders (IGAP) which was agreed in 2022 to run for ten years to address gaps in treatment, care and quality of life for all ages. The IGAP is not limited to epilepsy but includes other neurological disorders such as dementia, stroke, migraine and meningitis. In short, it focuses on brain health. An important aspect of the IGAP is that it was agreed at the global level by Member States of the WHO. Another aspect is that it includes carers and families not just people with neurological disorders. More importantly, carers and families, as well as civil society organisations and academics and the business sector were involved in creating the IGAP, making it people-centred. According to the ILAE, the IGAP addresses policy and governance; effective, timely and responsive diagnosis, treatment and care; promotion and prevention; research, innovation and information systems; and a public health response to epilepsy. The IGAP is the current global programme on epilepsy. It is too early to write about its impact, but not early to write about facilitators, opportunities, challenges and barriers.

Conclusion

A global response has many opportunities, but it presents challenges too. The major opportunity lies in the collaboration between countries, professionals and people with epilepsy and their families. Such collaboration facilitates the sharing of knowledge, expertise and resources, which can greatly enhance the effectiveness of epilepsy care worldwide. However, challenges persist, including issues of colonisation and dominance, particularly where the Global North exerts influence over the Global South. These challenges can affect how global policies and programmes are implemented and experienced in different regions. This chapter explored these dynamics by summarising key global organisations—WHO, ILAE, IBE and IBRO)—and their roles, discussing what constitutes policy and its importance, and outlining the policy-making process. It reviewed past and current global programmes on epilepsy and their implementation. This chapter also examines the roles of governments and communities, identifies policy gaps and suggests ways to address these issues to improve global responses to epilepsy.

References

Dos Santos, P. F., Cumbe, V., Gouveia, M. L., et al. (2019). Implementation of mhGAP in Mozambique: Integrating epilepsy care into the primary health care system. *International Journal of Mental Health Systems, 13*, 36. doi:10.1186/s13033-019-0296-5

International League Against Epilepsy (ILAE). (2008). *Global campaign against epilepsy.* Report. Dublin: ILAE.

International League Against Epilepsy (ILAE), International Bureau for Epilepsy (IBE) and World Health Organisation (WHO). (1997). *Global campaign against epilepsy.* Geneva: WHO

Kaculini, C. M., Tate-Looney, A. J., & Seifi, A. (2021). The history of epilepsy: From ancient mystery to modern misconception. *Cureus, 13*(3), e13953. doi:10.7759/cureus.13953

Li, L. M., Fernandes, P. T., de Boer, H. M., Prilipko, L., & Sander, J. W. (2007). Demonstration project on epilepsy in Brazil – WHO/ILAE/IBE global campaign against epilepsy: A foreword. *Arquivos de Neuro-Psiquiatria, 65*(suppl 1), 1–4. doi:10.1590/S0004-282X2007001000001

Min, L. L., & Sander, J. W. A. S. (2003). Projeto demonstrativo em epilepsia no Brasil. *Arquivos de Neuro-Psiquiatria, 61*(1), 153–156. doi:10.1590/S0004-282X2003000100033

Mugumbate, J. R. (2010). *Global campaign against epilepsy (GCAE) Zimbabwe report.* Harare: Epilepsy Support Foundation.

Mugumbate, R., Klevor R., Aguirre M. O., Massi G.D., Yaqoob N., Acevedo K., Yewnetu E., Kanyabutembo C., Ibrahim E. A. A., Boutadghart S., Janneh A., & Kissani N. (2023). Epilepsy awareness days, weeks, and months: Their roles in the fight against epilepsy and the intersectoral global action plan on epilepsy and other neurological disorders. *Epilepsy & Behavior, 148*, 109457, doi:10.1016/j.yebeh.2023.109457

Singh, G., Singh, M. B., Ding, D., Maulik, P., & Sander, J. W. (2023). Implementing WHO's Intersectoral Global Action Plan for epilepsy and other neurological disorders in Southeast Asia: A proposal. *The Lancet Regional Health. Southeast Asia, 10*, 100135. doi:10.1016/j.lansea.2022.100135

Wang, W., Wu, J., Bell, G. S., et al. (2008). Global campaign against epilepsy : Assessment of a demonstration project in rural China. *Bulletin of the World Health Organization, 86*(12), 964–969. doi:10.2471/BLT.07.047050

Wolf, P. (2002). Regional declarations and white papers. *Epilepsia, 43*(Suppl. 6), 37–43.

World Health Organization (WHO). (2002) *Mental health Global Action Programme: mhGAP.* Geneva: World Health Organization.

World Health Organization (WHO). (2004). *Atlas: Country resources for neurological disorders 2004.* Geneva: World Health Organization.

World Health Organization (WHO). (2007). *Neurological disorders: Public health challenges.* Geneva: World Health Organization.

World Health Organization (WHO). (2008) *mhGAP Mental Health Gap Action Programme. Scaling up care for mental, neurological, and substance use disorders.* Geneva: World Health Organization.

World Health Organization (WHO). (2015). *Declaration on the: Global burden of epilepsy and the need for coordinated action at the country level to address its health, social and public knowledge implications.* Geneva: World Health Organization.

Yang, H., Wen-zhi Wang W., Wu, J., et al (2012). Follow-up study of the WHO-Global Campaign Against Epilepsy Demonstration Project in rural China after four years of its termination. *Zhongguo Xian Dai Shen Jing Ji Bing Za Zhi, 12*(5), 530–535. doi:10.3969/j.issn.1672-6731.2012.05.007

10 Social work management strategies for epilepsy

There are multiple ways of socially managing epilepsy, and each gives different outcomes. This chapter discusses the values of social work, and the methods of casework, groupwork, community work, policy and international work used by social workers. The roles of social workers focussing on clinical, educational and community settings will also be discussed focussing on empowerment, participation and collaboration in interventions that are decolonial, contextual and culturally relevant. At the end, there will be an overview of other human service professions, including but not limited to counsellors, community workers, social scientists, social service professionals, human service workers, social welfare/welfare workers, Indigenous health workers, family workers, disability workers and village health workers. Social models have been used since time immemorial, however, newer social models continue to emerge but these are not used a lot in the Global South. The advantage with social models is that they are culturally constructed, and often acceptable.

The profession of social work

Social work is an academic programme, a profession and a service Africa Social Work and Development Network (ASWDNet, 2021). As an academic programme, social workers undergo training at college or university that culminates in a certificate, diploma or degree. The degrees include associate, bachelors, masters and doctoral. The profession is regulated at national and global levels. The basic social work training that is required to achieve a professional status includes theory, practice and in some instances, research (International Association of Schools of Social Work [IASSW], International Federation of Social Work [IFSW], & International Council of Social Welfare [ICSW], 2014). The fieldwork or placement involves students or trainee social workers spending several hours or months working with individuals, families, communities, groups and institutions to deliver social services under the supervision of a qualified social worker. Each country that has social work training has a national association of social workers, that acts as a labour union or a council that is a public body to regulate the profession (IASSW, IFSW, & ICSW, 2014). Other countries have both these, an association and a council, others have one entity that has all the labour and

DOI: 10.4324/9781003602866-10

regulatory roles. At the global level, the International Association of Schools of Social Work (IASSW) regulates training institutions, the International Federation of Social Workers (IFSW) is the labour union and the International Council of Social Welfare (ICSW) is the association of organisations and entities providing social welfare and services. There are also networks of social workers, including the Africa Social Work and Development Network (ASWDNet). As a service, social work is responsible for enraging, restoring and maintaining social functioning and development, and to ensure liberation, empowerment and justice. Before social work became an academic discipline and a profession, there were already people in each society mandated to provide social services. With time, social needs increased in society due to industrialisation, urbanisation, population growth and colonisation which disrupted the social fabrics of many communities in the Global South. In the Global North, one answer to these social challenges was to train social service workers and volunteers to be able to help more people, and this resulted in the social work profession. During colonisation, this approach was duplicated in colonised countries, most of them in the Global North, and this resulted in Eurocentric social work in the Middle East, Asia, the Pacific, the Caribbean, Latin America and Africa. The duplicated model included importing social workers from the Global North to work or train social workers in the Global South. Materials for teaching and learning all came from the Global North, so were the pedagogies. However, this type of social work had several loopholes, including that it was not suited to resource-poor settings where government funding for a welfare state is limited and more importantly, the social work developed in the Global North had a different cultural orientation which made it impossible to make an impact in the Global South, but rather contributed to colonisation. There have been several attempts to decolonise social work to make it more appropriate, for example, using decolonised literature produced locally or formation of networks such as the ASWDNet. In the Middle East, Asia, the Pacific, the Caribbean, Latin America and Africa, social work training institutions, academics, researchers and students are working to make social work more focused on the challenges on the ground, including epilepsy. Epilepsy requires a well thought out social management process because of different understandings of the condition, as illustrated in the previous chapters.

Information box 10.1   Definitions of social work

African definition of social work

Social work is an academic discipline and profession that embraces and enhances long-held methods of addressing life challenges in order to increase social functioning, development, cohesion and liberation using diverse Indigenous knowledges and values enshrined in the family, community, society, environment and in spirituality (ASWDNet, 2021).

Global definition of the social work profession

Social work is a practice-based profession and an academic discipline that promotes social change and development, social cohesion and the empowerment and liberation of people. Principles of social justice, human rights, collective responsibility and respect for diversities are central to social work. Underpinned by theories of social work, social sciences, humanities and Indigenous knowledges, social work engages people and structures to address life challenges and enhance well-being. The above definition may be amplified at national and/or regional levels (IASSW, IFSW, & ICSW, 2014).

Social work uses a strength and decolonising perspective that empowers and develops. The strengths perspective in social work focuses on the strengths and resources of individuals, families and communities instead of just their problems. These resources include their knowledge. This approach encourages social workers to identify and build on the positive qualities, skills and resilience of clients to help them overcome challenges and reach their goals. Using a strengths approach creates a more empowering and supportive relationship with clients. Disability organisations and the government should adopt a more open and strengths-based attitude. The strengths perspective shifts the focus from what is wrong to what is possible, leading to better outcomes in social work practice.

Goals of social management

The main goal of social work is to ensure, restore or maintain social functioning and social development, mainly following the social model of disability (Morgan, 2012; Mugumbate & Gray, 2016). In the context of managing epilepsy, specific goals and targets need to be put in place to ensure the implementation of effective strategies. The table below lists five goals and 17 targets to eradicate misconceptions and ongoing negative social attitudes about epilepsy and ensure: (i) medical treatment for all people with epilepsy, adequate work skills and employment positions for people with epilepsy, (ii) adequate and inclusive policies for people with epilepsy and (iii) adequate and inclusive services for people with epilepsy.

Information box 10.2   Social work with people with epilepsy

Goals	Targets
Eradicate misunderstandings and negative social attitudes about epilepsy (Mugumbate & Nyanguru, 2013).	Public health education and awareness to combat negative social attitudes focussing on family, school, workplace and community. Sensitisation of traditional healers and service providers.

Goals	Targets
Ensure medical treatment for all people with epilepsy (Mugumbate & Mushonga, 2013).	Access to medical treatment to ensure early control of seizures and streamlined epilepsy interventions to complement medical treatment.
Ensure adequate work skills and employment positions for people with disabilities (Mugumbate & Gray, 2021).	Basic education to enhance basic work skills. Increase the number of people with disabilities in vocational training to acquire work skills appropriate for the Zimbabwe job market. Job readiness programmes and employment services. Increase access to formal employment in the public and private sectors. Supportive employment workplace policies to ensure fairness in the workplace. Developmental approach that enhances opportunities within the informal sector.
Ensure adequate and inclusive policies for people with disability (Mugumbate & Gray, 2017a, 2017b).	Disability inclusion policies for all private, public and voluntary institutions and employers. Resource provision to create a positive supportive environment, including social assistance to facilitate employment access and retention. Inclusion of people with disabilities in policy-making structures to enhance voice and representation. Create legal channels for recourse to justice.
Ensure adequate and inclusive services for people with epilepsy (Mugumbate, Riphagenn, & Gathara, 2017).	Service provider capacity building to ensure quality service provision. Improve basic education, welfare and health services. Foster research in epilepsy and employment. Ensure adequate funding is available for services.

Roles of social workers in the managing of epilepsy

Mugumbate et al. (2017) studied the roles of social workers in the management of epilepsy and concluded that the roles are:

1 Psychosocial support and lifestyle management.
2 Enhancing service accessibility and resource mobilisation.
3 Employment issues and income maintenance.
4 Education and awareness raising.
5 Promoting the inclusion and participation of people with epilepsy.
6 Advocacy and lobbying.
7 Research and policy work.

The authors concluded their research by saying,

> Epilepsy remains an under-reported, under-recognised, under-treated, under-represented, under-resourced, and under-researched condition that presents multiple social challenges. Social workers have a role to deal with these 'u's in epilepsy. In managing these challenges, social workers must work with other professionals as part of a comprehensive developmental program that includes economic empowerment, medical therapy, psychosocial support, public education and awareness raising to reduce social stigma, increase treatment uptake, and promote treatment adherence. Further, they advocate and lobby for affordable and accessible treatment services, and research to inform public policy. A developmental approach that empowers people with epilepsy and addresses structural systemic factors that impede their potential to address the various medical, psychological, economic, cultural, and social challenges they face is thus needed.
>
> (Mugumbate et al., 2017)

In this chapter, the roles have been divided into direct practice, policy practice and research, developmental and international.

Direct practice roles

Direct practice roles played by social workers vary from country to country but include counselling, advocacy and family support. In Zimbabwe, social workers provide counselling and practical support for people in residential care (Chitereka, 2010; Jelsma, Mielke, Powell, De Weerdt, & De Cock, 2015). In addition to counselling, in other countries, social work roles in institutions include assessment, training, research and referrals, as shown in Table 10.1 (Beaulaurier & Taylor, 2001; Dhemba, 2011).

Table 10.1 Social work direct practice role

Role	Activities
Counselling	Conduct accurate assessments to identify needs, plan interventions and link people with services and benefits. Help people access direct funding, such as health insurance, pensions and other benefits, where these are available. Help people with disabilities plan for, and remain in, employment. Refer people to appropriate resources or services.
Advocacy	Reduce barriers and create pathways for vocational training. Improve access to primary, secondary and tertiary education for people with epilepsy by promoting school enrolment. Create access to healthcare.
Social and family support	Offer social and family support to manage the person with epilepsy, facilitate their social engagement and help them develop goals. Group work for psychosocial support. Engage in activities to raise community awareness to reduce stigma and discrimination.

In most countries, social workers work independently or as part of rehabilitation teams for people with disabilities that might include doctors, nurses, rehabilitation workers, advocators, counsellors, employment officers, welfare officers and teachers (Chitereka, 2010). Through direct practice, social workers ensure people's optimal social functioning by addressing the challenges hindering them from performing their social, economic, or political roles in society. They do this by conducting accurate assessments to identify needs, planning interventions and linking people with services and benefits, such as disability grants (Chitereka, 2010).

In Zimbabwe, social workers refer people to appropriate resources or services provided by government, non-government, private, or community-based organisations (Chitereka, 2010). Often, people with disabilities find it hard to navigate fragmented services, and face challenges in securing and completing vocational training, hence the need for advocacy (Mtetwa, 2011). Chitereka (2010) described how social workers in Lesotho facilitated vocational rehabilitation by assisting people with disabilities to make choices about courses, acquire assistive devices and gain skills.

Groupwork, or working with groups, is one of the ways in which social workers help people improve their social functioning. Its importance lies in its therapeutic, educative and social functions. It brings people together in groups, where they could share their experiences and speak freely in an accepting environment. In Zimbabwe, the Epilepsy Support Foundation (ESF) uses groupwork to train parents on seizure management, first aid, dealing with negative community attitudes and engage in income-generation ventures.

Policy practice and research

Through policy work, social workers promote human rights. The IFSW (2012) noted that social workers are directed and guided by the CRPD (United Nations [UN], 2006) in improving legislation, and developing and implementing just policies. They foster social inclusion, self-determination and freedom by highlighting inequalities and advocating for inclusive policies. Chitereka (2010) argued that policy work ensures effective social structures. Social workers advocate for the employment of people with disabilities in the public sector (Campbell, 2011). Labour-related advocacy includes promoting reasonable accommodation, open labour market participation and vocational and professional rehabilitation.

Research on disability is limited in Africa, especially Sub-Saharan Africa, especially on prevalence, challenges and opportunities (International Labour Organisation [ILO], 2007, 2008, 2013, 2015). This renders people with disabilities invisible and forgotten (ILO, 2008). Gray, Plath and Webb (2009) contend that social work practice should be informed by research, a view shared by the IFSW (2012). Research focused on issues surrounding disability, including opportunities, barriers, new technologies, and inclusion strategies and the employment experiences of people with disability (Campbell, 2011). Social workers carry out research to inform practice and contribute to the development of innovative, relevant and appropriate services (Chitereka, 2010). Their overall aim is to better understand disability and develop more effective approaches in reducing its impact. In African countries, like Zimbabwe, there is a need to keep abreast of new trends in disability work and to determine the applicability of strategies and interventions to local contexts. Jelsma et al. (2015) conceded that there had been very little research on disability intervention.

Developmental practice

African countries have seen a shift towards developmental social work, which is viewed as empowering (Mupedziswa, 2001; Mupedziswa & Kubanga, 2016). Developmental social work sought culturally, socially and economically appropriate approaches (Gray & Ariong, 2017). It addressed unjust structural disadvantages (Hall, 1990; Mupedziswa & Kubanga, 2016) and sought preventive solutions (Mupedziswa & Sinkamba, 2014) and increased income for the poor (Mhiribidi, 2010). Table 10.2 outlines the goals of developmental social work that seeks change at the individual, community and national levels.

At the individual level, developmental social work seeks to build human capital through education and training, employment and microenterprise development (Gathiram, 2008). At the community level, it seeks to enhance participation and give people a voice in development and increase access to services. At the national level, it seeks policies to address structural inequality by developing accessible markets for goods and services through multisectoral programmes, including sustainable social security. In these ways, developmental social work aims to remove structural barriers to development.

Within developmental social work, community development involves raising awareness and mobilising resources to enhance employment opportunities (Chitereka, 2010; Jelsma et al., 2015). In economies like Zimbabwe, where opportunities for formal employment are limited, social workers engage in projects to provide opportunities for self-employment, entrepreneurship, cooperative

Table 10.2 Developmental social work roles

Level	Strategy
Individual	Enhance human capital, that is, individual knowledge and skills through education and training.
	Make employment accessible, that is, create jobs.
	Initiate sustainable microenterprises, that is, family and community-owned businesses.
Community	Enhance community participation in development.
	Enhance access to, and use of, community services.
National	Develop policies to address structural inequality and socioeconomic disadvantage, such as employment creation.
	Ensure sustainable development for long-term change.
	Develop accessible markets for goods and services.
	Ensure planned multisectoral programmes.
	Make social security viable.

engagement and business ownership (Mpofu & Harley, 2002; Mugumbate et al., 2017).

Social workers play an important role in coordinating disability programmes, linking people with schools, churches, community leaders and civil society organisations (Mugumbate et al., 2017). They provide information, share experiences, and offer training services, create partnerships with service users, providers and the community based on the belief that people with disabilities would be more socially and economically productive if community transport, housing, education and health services were more accessible (Oliver, 2013).

Gray (2010) highlighted that these developmental goals sustained the *status quo* within neoliberal welfare systems. Nevertheless, developmental social work implies a service continuum, starting with building human capital through the creation of a supportive family and community environment, and instituting policies and programmes to ensure that people with disabilities have access to the social goods and services they need to lead full and productive lives, that is, food, health, education, work, shelter, physical security and participation. Developmental social work advocated an integrated approach including people with disabilities in mainstream service provision, education and employment or economic participation and hence makes the community an important locus for disability programmes. Social workers work with communities to take responsibility for their development through empowering programmes that help people to manage their own lives and remain independent (Gray, 2010; Mupedziswa & Kubanga, 2016). Communities are reservoirs of social capital with social workers harnessing and building on individual and group strengths for targeted intervention programmes. Ultimately, the aim of developmental social work and disability work is social justice.

International social work

When social workers work across borders, this becomes international social work. Working across borders includes collaborating with social workers from other countries, managing epilepsy in other countries, funding programmes or volunteering in other countries or developing policies that can be used in more than one country. A specific example of an international social work group in epilepsy is the Social Work and Social Services Section of the International league Against Epilepsy (ILAE). The group is made up of social workers, counsellors, community workers, social scientists, social service professionals, human service workers and Indigenous and cultural health workers all play vital roles in supporting individuals and communities. There professionals in this group provide services that address various social, emotional, economic and cultural needs, helping to promote well-being and enhance the quality of life for those they serve. The group's objectives include creating a communication platform and resources for social workers who work with epilepsy, assessing the learning and practice needs of social workers around the world, and developing educational programmes that can be tailored to different regions. They aim to encourage social workers to take part in ILAE councils and committees, and to be involved in educating healthcare professionals and the public. Additionally, the group wants to improve communication, knowledge sharing, and networking among social work and neurology professionals globally. They will also mentor students and junior social workers, support other ILAE sections, and provide expertise in social science research and evaluation.

Other professions and role players in the managing of epilepsy

Counsellors are important in managing epilepsy, especially in resource-limited settings, as they provide emotional support to individuals and their families. They help people deal with feelings like anxiety and fear that often accompany the condition. In their sessions, they teach coping strategies and offer information about epilepsy, which can significantly improve mental well-being.

Community workers play a key role in raising awareness about epilepsy in resource-limited settings. They work to reduce stigma by organising educational programmes and workshops that inform people about the condition. For instance, the Peruvian Association of Epilepsy conducts outreach initiatives to educate communities and dispel myths surrounding the disorder. In Lebanon, the Avance Association of People with Epilepsy and Special Needs focuses on providing support and resources for individuals with epilepsy. The Nepal Epilepsy Association also works to promote awareness and offer support services. In South Korea, the Korea Bureau for Epilepsy actively raises awareness and provides educational resources to help people understand epilepsy better. Additionally, Epilepsy Fiji is active in educating the public and providing assistance to those affected by epilepsy, ensuring they have access to care and information. In Sierra Leone, the Epilepsy Association works tirelessly to support individuals with epilepsy and their families, helping to create a more inclusive environment. These community efforts help individuals connect with resources, support groups and healthcare services.

Social scientists contribute by conducting research that helps improve policies and practices related to epilepsy in resource-limited settings. They study the social and cultural issues that affect people with the condition and identify barriers to care. Their findings can lead to better access to healthcare and support services. When they analyse trends and data, social scientists provide insights that can shape public health initiatives and enhance the lives of individuals with epilepsy.

Social service professionals coordinate care for people with epilepsy in resource-limited environments. They assess the needs of patients and their families, connecting them with resources like healthcare and financial support. They advocate for their clients, ensuring they receive the help they need to manage their condition. They guide individuals through complex systems and help them access essential services that improve their quality of life.

Human service workers provide direct support to individuals with epilepsy in resource-limited settings. They assist clients in creating and following personal care plans tailored to their needs. These workers often collaborate with other professionals, such as healthcare providers and educators, to build a strong support network. Their practical approach ensures that individuals receive the help they need to manage their condition and lead fulfilling lives.

Indigenous and cultural health workers offer culturally sensitive care to individuals with epilepsy, particularly in resource-limited settings. They understand the unique challenges faced by Indigenous communities and combine traditional healing practices with modern medicine. For example, Aboriginal health workers in Australia engage with Indigenous people living with epilepsy, respecting their cultural beliefs and practices. Similarly, health workers supporting the Sidi people in Asia incorporate cultural understanding and traditional approaches into their care. Health workers engage effectively with individuals and families, which helps improve health outcomes and fosters a sense of belonging for those with epilepsy.

Family workers play a crucial role in supporting individuals with epilepsy providing guidance and resources to families. They help families understand the condition, how to manage it, and how to give emotional support to their loved ones. Drawing on ideas like Confucianism, which emphasises family harmony and respect, and Hindu beliefs that value community support, family workers encourage strong family connections. They also use Buddhist principles of compassion and mindfulness to help families cope with stress and anxiety related to epilepsy. Additionally, Ubuntu philosophy highlights the importance of community and interconnectedness, reminding families that they are not alone in their journey. Family workers facilitate communication between family members and healthcare providers, ensuring that everyone knows about treatment plans and care strategies. They also assist families in accessing community resources and services, helping them navigate challenges related to employment, education and social support. By creating a supportive environment at home, informed by these philosophies, family workers contribute to the overall well-being of individuals with epilepsy.

Disability workers focus on empowering individuals with epilepsy, promoting their rights and ensuring they have access to necessary services. They work to create inclusive environments where individuals can participate fully in society, whether in education, employment, or social activities. Disability workers assess the specific needs of individuals and connect them with appropriate resources, such as therapy, counselling and vocational training. They advocate for policy changes that improve accessibility and support for people with disabilities, using the social model of disability and the WHO model, which highlights the interaction between health conditions and environmental factors. They also consider the UN model of disability, which stresses the importance of human rights and social inclusion. This approach shows that barriers in society, rather than the impairment itself, create challenges for individuals. Raising awareness about the difficulties faced by people with epilepsy, disability workers help reduce stigma and promote a more inclusive community.

Village health workers can work closely with village leaders and local kings or rulers by involving them in awareness campaigns and health education efforts. For instance, in Jamaica, the Jamaican Epilepsy Association engages village health workers to promote understanding and support within communities. Similarly, the Community Development and Epilepsy Foundation in Cameroon collaborates with local leaders to raise awareness about epilepsy. These respected figures can help reduce stigma and encourage community support for affected individuals. By partnering with village leaders, health workers can organise health fairs and workshops to educate the public about epilepsy, addressing cultural beliefs and misconceptions. Additionally, local rulers can advocate for better healthcare resources and policies that improve access to treatment for those with epilepsy. This collaboration creates a stronger support system within the community, benefiting both individual health and overall community well-being.

Conclusion

Social work is a professional skill that is acquired through years of training and improved through experience. This chapter discussed the role of social work in the management of epilepsy. These roles are played at different levels—the individual, family, community, societal and international levels to bring, restore or maintain social functioning and development. There is no doubt that social work plays a significant role in the management of epilepsy; however, in most resource-poor settings, social work is non-existent or exists in urban communities. Even where social workers exist, they are in short supply that conditions such as epilepsy are rarely prioritised or the social workers do not have the skills to practice in the local context because of irrelevant training. These challenges can be addressed by training more social workers using a decolonised curriculum that responds to local needs and priorities.

References

Africa Social Work and Development Network (ASWDNet). (2021). African definition of the Social Work Profession. Retrieved from https://africasocialwork.net/

Beaulaurier, R., & Taylor, S. (2001). Social work practice with people with disabilities in the era of disability rights. *Social Work Health Care, 32*(4), 67–91.

Campbell, F. K. (2011). *The NDIS—A pathway to employment?* Paper presented at the Australia's Disability Employment Services Conference, Brisbane, June 29, 2011.

Chitereka, C. (2010). People with disabilities and the role of Social Workers in Lesotho. *Social Work and Society International Online Journal, 8*(1). Online.

Dhemba, J. (2011). People with disabilities and the role of social workers in Lesotho. *Social Work and Society, 8*(1), 82–93.

Gathiram, N. (2008). A critical review of the developmental approach to disability in South Africa. *International Journal of Social Welfare, 17*(2), 146–155.

Gray, M. (2010). Social development and the status quo: Professionalisation and Third Way cooptation. *International Journal of Social Welfare, 19*(4), 463–470.

Gray, M., & Ariong, S. B. (2017). Discourses shaping development, foreign aid, and poverty reduction policies in Africa: Implications for social work. In M. Gray (Ed.), *The handbook of social work and social development in Africa* (pp. 15–32). London: Routledge.

Gray, M., Plath, D., & Webb, S. A. (2009). *Evidence-based social work: A critical stance.* London: Routledge.

Hall, N. (1990). *Social work training in Africa: A fieldwork manual.* Harare: School of Social Work.

International Association of Schools of Social Work (IASSW), International Federation of Social Work (IFSW), & International Council of Social Welfare (ICSW). (2014). Global definition of the Social Work Profession. Retrieved from https://www.ifsw.org/what-is-social-work/global-definition-of-social-work/

International Federation of Social Workers (IFSW). (2012). *People with disabilities.* Retrieved July 20, 2016. from https://ifsw.org/policies/people-with-disabilities/

International Labour Organisation (ILO). (2007). *Skills development through Community Based Rehabilitation (CBR). A good practice guide.* Geneva: ILO.

International Labour Organisation (ILO). (2008). Employment and disabled persons information sheet.

International Labour Organisation (ILO). (2013). *Inclusion of people with disabilities in Zambia.* Lusaka: ILO.

International Labour Organisation (ILO). (2015). *Disability inclusion strategy and action plan 2014–17.* Geneva: ILO.

Jelsma, J., Mielke, J., Powell, G., De Weerdt, W., & De Cock, P. (2015). Disability in an urban black community in Zimbabwe. *Disability & Rehabilitation, 24*(16), 851–859.

Mhiribidi, S. T. W. (2010). Promoting the developmental social welfare approach in Zimbabwe: Challenges and prospects. *Journal of Social Development in Africa, 25*(2), 121–146.

Morgan, H. (2012). The social model of disability as a threshold concept: Troublesome knowledge and liminal spaces in social work education. *Social Work Education, 31*(2), 215–226.

Mpofu, E. & Harley, D. A. (2002). Disability and rehabilitation in Zimbabwe: Lessons and implications for rehabilitation practice in the U.S. *Journal of Rehabilitation; Alexandria, 68*(4), 26–33.

Mtetwa, E. (2011). Policy dimensions of exclusion: Disability as charity and not right in Zimbabwe. *Indian Journal of Social Work, 72*(3), 381–398.

Mugumbate, J., & Gray, M. (2016). Social justice and disability policy in Southern Africa. *Journal of Social Development in Africa, 31*(2), 7–24.

Mugumbate, J., & Gray, M. (2017a). Competing traditional and medical treatments of epilepsy in Harare, Zimbabwe. *African and Middle East Journal of Epilepsy* (accepted for publication).

Mugumbate, J., & Gray, M. (2017b). Individual resilience as a strategy to counter employment barriers for people with epilepsy in Zimbabwe. *Epilepsy and Behaviour, 74C*, 154–160. March. doi:10.1016/j.yebeh.2017.06.018

Mugumbate, J., & Gray, M. (2021). Employment rights for people with epilepsy in Zimbabwe: A social justice perspective. In V. Sewpaul, L. Kreitzer, & T. Raniga (Ed.), *Culture, human rights and social work: African perspectives,* (pp. 81–99). Calgary: University of Calgary.

Mugumbate, J., & Mushonga, J. (2013). Myths, perceptions, and incorrect knowledge surrounding epilepsy in rural Zimbabwe: A study of the villagers in Buhera District. *Epilepsy and Behavior, 27*(1), 144–147.

Mugumbate, J., & Nyanguru, A. (2013). Measuring the challenges of people with epilepsy in Harare, Zimbabwe. *Neurology Asia, 18*(1), 29–33.

Mugumbate, J., Riphagenn, H., & Gathara, R. (2017). The role of social workers in the social management of epilepsy in Africa. In M. Gray (Ed.), *The handbook of social work and social development in Africa* (pp. 168–180). London: Routledge.

Mupedziswa, R. (2001). The quest for relevance: Towards a conceptual model of developmental social work education and training in Africa. *International Social Work, 44*(3), 285–300.

Mupedziswa, R., & Kubanga, K. (2016). Developing social work education in Africa: Challenges and prospects. In I. Taylor, M. Bogo, M. Lefevre, & B. Teater (Eds.), *Routledge international handbook of social work education* (pp. 119–130). London: Routledge.

Mupedziswa, R., & Sinkamba, R. (2014). Social work education and training in Southern and East Africa: Yesterday, today and tomorrow. In H. S. C. Noble & B. Littlechild (Eds.), *Global social work: Crossing borders, blurring boundaries* (pp 141–154). Sydney: Sydney University Press.

Oliver, M. (2013). *The social model of disability: Thirty years on* (vol. 28). Oxfordshire: Carfax International Publishers.

Rutsate, S. (2009). Engaging interventions of vocational rehabilitation. *International Journal of Disability, Development and Education, 56*(2), 183–188. doi:10.1080/10349120902868640

United Nations (UN). (2006). *Convention on the rights of persons with disabilities*. New York: UN.

11 Building and sustaining resilience

Maintaining family and individual resilience is crucial in managing epilepsy, a key theme highlighted by a study conducted in Zimbabwe. Resilience refers to the ability to adapt and bounce back from challenges or difficulties, and in the context of epilepsy, it means being able to handle the condition's impact on daily life and relationships effectively. The study from Zimbabwe showed that resilience in both individuals and their families plays a significant role in managing epilepsy. This resilience helps people cope with the emotional, social and practical challenges that come with the condition. The findings from this study are not just relevant to Zimbabwe but have important implications for other parts of the world where people face similar challenges. The first part of this chapter will explore what resilience means and why it is important for managing epilepsy. This will be followed by a detailed look at how the Zimbabwe study was carried out, including the methods used to gather and analyse data. Finally, this chapter will summarise the key results of the study, showing how the findings can help improve understanding and support for people with epilepsy everywhere.

The nature of resilience

Epilepsy impacts the ability of individuals and their families to cope with life challenges (WHO, 2016; Saburi, 2011). This is because it is unpredictable and often the management is life-long. There are also high levels of stigma attached to the condition. Studies have shown the importance of individual resilience in people with epilepsy (Richardson, 2002; Munn, 2008; Day, 2008; Ring, Jacob, Baker, Marson, & Whitehead, 2016). A number of studies showed that resilience helped people with epilepsy to adapt to, or survive, adversity associated with debilitating seizures and socioeconomic disadvantage and have a good quality of life (Day, 2008; Ring et al., 2016) aided by fewer side effects of treatment and the absence of depression (Taylor et al., 2011). Resilience facilitated employment but its absence meant that some people with epilepsy were vulnerable to biopsychosocial disruption (Ring et al., 2016). Advocates of the resiliency model argued that individuals experienced biopsychosocial disruption after which they reintegrated in a manner that improved their quality of life and reduced their vulnerability (Richardson, 2002).

DOI: 10.4324/9781003602866-11

Other studies showed that self-management was an important characteristic of resilient individuals. Resilient individuals depended on their psychological self-management abilities, such as resource seeking, acceptance of epilepsy and environmental resources, including patient support networks, the positive attitudes of employers or co-workers or strong family support (Ring et al., 2016). Resilient self-managers controlled their epilepsy by seeking and maintaining treatment (Munn, 2008). Seizure frequency had no significant impact on the quality of life of resilient individuals (Day, 2008). This showed that better employment outcomes were achieved by those who were resilient despite seizures.

Prior research suggested that service providers were encouraged to integrate resilience-building factors into standard care practices (Ring et al., 2016; Edward, Cook & Giandinoto, 2015), including helping people with epilepsy build psychological self-management strategies to cope with adversity (Taylor et al., 2011). It acknowledged that resilience could be only part of standard care practices, meaning that service providers did not need to rely solely on individual resilience to achieve better employment outcomes.

Methodology of the Zimbabwe study

The study site was the Epilepsy Support Foundation (ESF) in Harare, Zimbabwe's main urban area and capital. The ESF provides access to epilepsy treatment, psychosocial support, economic empowerment, disability advocacy and awareness-raising services. Specific interventions at the ESF include counselling, support groups, information centre, dispensary, electroencephalogram (EEG) diagnosis, income-generating projects and epilepsy awareness through inter alia National Epilepsy Awareness Week, International Epilepsy Day, Purple Day and the distribution of literature and information dissemination. The ESF was selected as a study site because it provided researchers with easy access to its service users and service providers being the only support organisation for people with epilepsy in the country. People with epilepsy in Zimbabwe often do not disclose their condition and it is difficult for researchers to identify them, except through institutions providing them with services, such as the ESF.

This chapter reports on data from eight participants, who were classified as resilient, out of 30 participants who took part in the in-depth interviews. The eight resilient participants comprised four males and four females whose ages ranged from 26 to 48 years. They had overcome chronic unemployment. Seven were employed while one had recently become unemployed. The eight participants were receiving medical treatment and described their seizures as controlled (n = 2), partially controlled (n = 3) and fully controlled (n = 3). Four participants had experienced their first seizures during childhood and four during adulthood. The demographic characteristics of participants are presented in Table 11.1. Pseudonyms were used to ensure the anonymity of participants, while names of actual occupations were avoided in favour of more generic descriptive terms. Other demographic information, such as marital status, were also removed to ensure anonymity.

Table 11.1 Social demographic characteristics of participants

Participant	Characteristics
Resilient female participants (n = 4)	
Saru	A 39-year-old government worker. Worked at three different schools, dismissed at one school because of epilepsy. Adult onset fully controlled epilepsy.
Mucha	A 32-year-old government worker. Childhood onset partially controlled epilepsy.
Grace	A 48-year-old government worker in a public hospital. Dismissed from a similar job during internship. Teenage onset-controlled epilepsy.
Tindo	A 33-year-old who was unemployed. Held a diploma. Worked in retail shops before but was underpaid and felt underrated. Adult onset-controlled epilepsy.
Resilient male participants (n = 4)	
Munya	A 33-year-old bank worker with a university degree and other qualifications. Missed a lucrative job opportunity after having seizures during probation. Dismissed from other jobs before due to seizures. Adult onset fully controlled epilepsy.
Lameck	A 28-year-old technician. Contract not renewed at an immediate past job. Adult onset fully controlled epilepsy.
Edson	A 26-year-old customer care worker. No ordinary level passes or any other qualifications. Not secure at present job because of seizures. Childhood onset with partially controlled seizures.
Farai	A 32-year-old maintenance worker. Did not pass ordinary levels and an apprenticeship course. Childhood onset partially controlled.

To supplement the in-depth interview data, a focus group discussion was conducted with service providers (n = 7) employed by the ESF. The service providers included three social service workers, two health workers and two disability advocacy workers. It was important to include service providers for two reasons. First, to focus their attention on employment issues, not usually a major preoccupation of their support work and, secondly, to get their opinions on the experiences of people with epilepsy with whom they worked.

A semi-structured interview guide was used with people with epilepsy, while a focus group discussion guide was used with service providers. Service providers were first presented with a summarised report of findings from the in-depth interviews, which they read before the focus group discussion. Data collection involved audio recording of responses from people with epilepsy and service providers. The data was then transcribed verbatim. These two data sets were analysed separately using NVivo, a computer-assisted qualitative data-analysis package. The analysis sought to understand the common and exceptional experiences of participants and how these experiences influenced their employment prospects. To achieve this, the transcripts were read several times to gain familiarisation with the data. Emerging codes were noted and the researcher added a few codes he had developed during fieldwork. The resultant codes were then loaded into NVivo to form initial codes that identified broad themes around experiences, barriers and facilitators. Individual resilience was one of the themes. The next section presents the barriers to employment, experiences of resilience and opinions of service providers.

Lessons from the Zimbabwe study

Barriers were encountered during job seeking

Participants' experiences showed that lack of educational qualifications was a barrier to job seeking. Hence, participants like Grace, Tindo, Lameck, Edson and Farai could not apply for jobs because they were underqualified. Asked why she did not have adequate educational qualifications, Grace said she had challenges acquiring basic education:

> Epilepsy started in 1984 when I was at boarding school, [school name removed]. I stopped going to school … [when I resumed] I did not go back to boarding school. I went to a local school.

Grace withdrew temporarily from school but later continued, though at a school with poorer facilities. Grace said her family had not fully supported her education at the well-resourced boarding school believing she would not be accepted there or would not succeed because of her epilepsy. She had to sit the examinations several times to pass the five subjects required for a tertiary qualification. This affected her job seeking because most companies preferred candidates who had passed the examinations in the first sitting. Grace intended to train as a teacher or nurse to get a diploma, but the training colleges required candidates who had passed the examination the first-time round. By the time of the interviews, she had not secured training and was past the age limit set by most training colleges. However, she trained as a non-skilled worker, obtained a certificate and got a job, but this was not the qualification or job she had desired.

Participants said delayed seizure control was another major reason why their education and training were not strong. All participants—Saru, Mucha, Grace, Tindo, Munya, Lameck, Edson and Farai—reported challenges with acquiring initial medical treatment, mainly because of the dominance of traditional and religious knowledge and beliefs geared towards non-medical treatment services. Resultantly, misunderstanding of epilepsy led to delayed treatment, which, in turn, led to poor educational and training outcomes.

Tindo and Grace reported that they had no access to government employment support services and, although they had relied on nongovernment organisations, such as the ESF and Ruwa Rehabilitation Centre, they had not received adequate employment services to assist with writing resumes, interview coaching, referral letters and career guidance. Grace reported that there were few jobs available in the open labour market, largely due to Zimbabwe's failed economy. This increased competition and, without support services, she was greatly disadvantaged.

Tindo and Mucha reported that they faced challenges in the home that prevented them from successful job seeking. They were both married. In the case of Tindo, her husband did not allow her to look for a job, fearing that she would face challenges in the workplace. Mucha said, 'my husband is very supportive'. Mucha's challenges were that she had more chores at home and this impacted on her work, since she was already employed.

Farai and Edson said, although they were employed, they faced the challenge of having few social contacts necessary for job seeking. Farai said he had lost most of his friends when his seizures began. Farai's brother got work at his father's workplace, but Farai could not because of his condition. Farai was later employed by an organisations, where he had volunteered for about a year, while a relative had helped Edson to secure a job. Edson had not disclosed his condition, while Farai did.

Job seekers often did probation or work-related learning. While on three-month's probation, Munya had had three seizures at work and did not get the job. He said that, in normal circumstances, people were employed by the company following probation; given that he had worked so well, he had expected an appointment but was unsuccessful due to his epilepsy. Grace was on work-related learning when she had a seizure and her contract was terminated instantly. Saru, Mucha, Lameck and Edson said they had been able to get jobs because they had not disclosed; they were afraid that once they disclosed their epilepsy, they would lose their jobs or be treated differently.

Barriers were encountered in the workplace

In the workplace, Lameck, Edson and Saru encountered negative attitudes from managers and co-workers once they knew about their epilepsy. Tindo and Lameck had experienced unfavourable employment conditions followed by dismissal from work. Farai, Lameck and Mucha reported that their employers feared that they would die at work or scare off customers. Edson reported that co-workers had doubted his capacity and 'disagreed when management gave him the worker of the month award'. Saru, Munya and Tindo were each dismissed from four jobs, while Mucha, Grace and Ashley had been dismissed from two jobs because of their condition. Edson and Farai had each been dismissed once. Despite discrimination in the workplace, there was no recourse to justice because participants had no hope of winning the cases of discrimination in court, and lacked the resources for litigation.

Participants said employers had treated them unfairly once they had disclosed their epilepsy. While Edson had not disclosed his condition to his employer, Lameck and Munya had disclosed but their employers had not supported them, since they 'viewed epilepsy as a spiritual rather than a health condition'. Lameck was not allowed time off to seek treatment, while Munya had been dismissed for spending a lot of time off work. Lameck had been 'transferred from department to department' and had been denied responsibilities at the factory where he worked 'because they thought I would die at work'. Edson said he had not been 'taken seriously at work'. At times, supervisors had brushed off Lameck in favour of 'the next guy'. He added:

> I think the way they took it they did not have full knowledge. They were not informed. Management was saying I could die at work or have another seizure. I would feel the segregation when duties were shared but I could feel that I could do this and that.

Although Lameck had explained his situation, his contract had not been renewed. He had looked for another job and had not disclosed his condition. In his new job, he had worked from the top of construction scaffolds, something that he had feared, but had to do because he had no other option. He had then enrolled in a diploma course in preparation for leaving the construction job due to his discomfort with it. Tindo, too, had faced several challenges, as illustrated in the case vignette of Tindo.

> Tindo was 33-years old by the time of the study. Her epilepsy started when she was already a young adult. She had completed her secondary education but had not passed all the subjects required to proceed to high school or college. Her family pursued traditional treatments and only embraced medical treatment after four years. Tindo and her family faced negative attitudes, such as stigma from the community. She faced several challenges when she married and the marriage did not last. Some of the challenges had to do with gender roles and her husband's refusal to allow her to work. After the failure of her marriage, she had looked unsuccessfully for work, even though she had acquired a diploma. She was unable to get any government or non-government employment support services. She eventually found work in a retail shop. The owner knew about her condition but was willing to hire her, though she was underpaid, despite having been dependable. She thought this would improve but did not. She approached the employer, who indicated that she had hired her because of her condition and that no one else would hire her. Frustrated, she had resigned and another company had hired her. She believed she was hired because of her impressive work performance at her prior workplace. Sadly, this new company had gone out of business and she was jobless once again. By the time of the study, Tindo had enrolled in a diploma program at a local college.

Tindo's experience showed most of the barriers she and her fellow participants encountered, including a lack of education and delayed seizure control. Without employment support services, participants like Tindo resorted to self-management. Despite these barriers, all eight participants overcame chronic unemployment and had not abandoned hope of achieving better employment outcomes. Their resilience was characterised by a 'fighting spirit'. They had been their own advocates and had mastered their epilepsy, as discussed in the following three sections.

People with epilepsy adopted a 'fighting spirit'

Participants adopted a 'fighting spirit' in society and in the workplace. Acquiring the education and skills needed for jobs was extremely challenging for all eight participants. However, Munya had a university degree and was enrolled in a professional course to improve his chances at his workplace. His epilepsy began during his final year at university, and he had overcome the pressures this put on him. He had acquired a driver's licence, despite the lengthy process due to his condition, and had remained positive, as his story of resilience presented in the case vignette of Munya.

> Munya's seizures had begun during his final year of university. The immediate explanation was that he had been bewitched to prevent him from graduating. As a result, his family had sought traditional interventions but these had not stopped his seizures. Munya could have dropped out of university but he had not. After graduating, he got a part-time job at the company where he had done his internship, but had been dismissed due to his seizures. He was not on medical treatment and had been taken to the hospital several times following seizures but had only received attention for injuries. He had not been properly diagnosed. He got a job at a parastatal (semi-government institution), where he was put on three-months' probation. During the period, he had had two seizures at work and had not got the job. He said he was surprised because he had worked exceptionally well. As was the norm in Zimbabwe, due to a weak economy, Munya went to neighbouring country, Namibia, to find work. He found a job and worked well, remaining seizure free. The job in Namibia required him to have a driver's licence so he had gone back to Zimbabwe to get one. He could not get the licence because he needed to be seizure free for at least two years. He could not go back to Namibia. Luckily, he attended an interview and got a job at a company he had worked with before. In his opinion, the main reason he got the job was that he had shown them that, despite his epilepsy, he was hard working and highly productive. He sought medical treatment at ESF and his seizures were reduced. After two years, he applied successfully for his driver's licence and was allowed to drive company vehicles at his new workplace. He became an active member of ESF. By the time of the study, he was enrolled for a professional course to enhance his promotion prospects at work.

Munya's story showed the challenges he faced and the strategies he employed to overcome them. His story corroborated that of other participants. Similarly, Lameck and Tindo had enrolled in diploma programmes to enhance their employment chances. Grace had moved from office to office, pestering government officials to provide her with a place to train or a job. She had finally found employment at a government hospital. At the time of the study, she was still pestering them to provide her with college training so she could become a skilled worker. Mucha too showed that it was important to develop a positive attitude. He said a 'fighting spirit' was needed. Such a positive attitude to their seemingly hopeless situation allowed some participants to overcome employment barriers. In the workplace, participants like Tindo and Edson had proved that they were hard workers. Due to her hard work, Tindo had gained her employer's trust quickly, while Edson had been crowned worker of the month for his diligence.

Female participants, such as Saru and Mucha, had experienced challenges balancing work at home and their jobs. They often felt overwhelmed. Saru said duties at home usually impacted on her work. Mucha said that, being a female worker, wife and person with a chronic condition was:

> The boring aspect of epilepsy, especially for women like myself, is that after work you need to work at home again. You then need to sleep early and prepare for work again. At times, I feel like I should start my own company and control my timetable.

Mucha's argument was that, with so many chores to do at home, she was deprived of the rest time needed before work the next day. Her employer was not flexible and she had contemplated self-employment so she would be able to control her work time.

People with epilepsy became their own advocates

Edson and Munya said people with epilepsy must act as advocates for sound employment policies. Munya noted:

> I told my boss I have epilepsy. That is me. If you ask me to raise a policy [part of his job] I will do that. If you give me any job, I will do it. If I have a seizure in front of a client and you lost business, then I am sorry but that is my situation.

Munya, who could be interviewed at work, had faced several challenges in the past, but thought the best way was for people with epilepsy to challenge society to understand and accommodate them.

Other participants showed that it was important to be their own advocates. Tindo had unsuccessfully challenged her employer for underpaying her. Edson had challenged his co-workers for labelling him a 'Sascam', a derogatory term referring to a person with low intelligence unable to take care of themselves. At work, Saru insisted that she be given equal duties to her co-workers, because she could work just as effectively as they could without epilepsy.

People with epilepsy developed mastery of the condition

The eight participants had been clear about their treatment, side effects and the need for compliance with medication. Edson, Munya and Mucha's experiences showed that mastering and accepting epilepsy was necessary to achieve better employment outcomes. Asked to share experiences that improved his outcomes, Edson said:

> In most cases, I think it starts with you, the person with epilepsy. You should accept your condition and educate people around you. Know what your condition requires. If you educate someone and they do not understand, ask someone else who knows to further educate them.

Mucha said she had been able to comply with medical treatment and take charge of her situation:

> Get yourself treated, maintain yourself so that you can keep your work. Those not employed, do self-jobs like woodwork, welding, and just do not neglect yourself. Epilepsy is just a condition.

Asked to explain, Mucha said that she had been mindful of her treatment and had controlled the factors that could trigger her seizures. Saru had accepted her condition and complied with medical treatment. Farai, too, had been cognisant of triggering factors, such as sun heat, and often discussed these with his supervisor.

Service providers agreed with the barriers and resilience

When asked for their opinion on the work experiences of participants, the service providers agreed that people with epilepsy faced challenges in education and this affected their employment opportunities. Service provider 5, an advocacy officer, blamed the education system for the situation of people with epilepsy, saying society labelled them as incapable and limited their educational opportunities:

> Those [people with epilepsy] who excel through it's either by force or by God's grace. If you look at the environment at schools, it's not conducive for a person with epilepsy. One, teachers are not equipped to handle children with epilepsy. As an example, at one school the headmaster told the parents 'take away your child; bring child when better'. What does that mean? Where will she take that child? You see, hence, it's just a way in which the system is discriminating against the person with epilepsy....

This meant that success for people with epilepsy was difficult as they encountered several barriers. Service provider 5 said it was always important to have schoolteachers and headmasters who knew how to deal with children with epilepsy. He recommended improved teacher training. However, Service provider 3, a health worker, thought the parents were to blame for their children's poor education:

> The parents will say you are wasting our time, you can't proceed with school. They (people with epilepsy) are asked to sit at home doing nothing. But they

forget the person is taking medication, and is able to proceed with school. But they blame the person saying you are failing school, yet it's because of seizures.

Service providers agreed that a lack of adequate medical treatment affected employment in several ways. They bemoaned the delays in receiving medical treatment and the lack of effective medical treatment services the interview participants had experienced but said this was a usual occurrence. Service provider 5 said many people with epilepsy delayed medical treatment as they did not know that epilepsy was a treatable condition: 'There is lack of knowledge within communities'. Service providers 1 and 4 agreed, adding that health centres did not usually have an adequate supply of antiepilepsy medicines and most lacked nurses trained to manage epilepsy, the unavailability of doctors notwithstanding. Although services were much better in urban areas, they were still basic and unaffordable for many, hence the attraction of the ESF. They seemed to agree that epilepsy was neglected both as a disability and a chronic health condition. Service providers 1 and 7 agreed that health services were poor, with an undersupply of medicines and inadequate personnel.

Focus group participants agreed with interview participants that self-management was important for improving employment opportunities. Service providers 1 and 3 emphasised that people with epilepsy needed the skills to manage their treatment, epilepsy triggers and the side effects of medication or this would impact on their ability to work. Service provider 3 said issues encountered included work events or stresses that triggered seizures, such as the over use of computers or loud noises, the side effects of medication that made them dizzy and ineffective treatments.

Service providers agreed that there was negativity and doubt in the workplace once it was known they had epilepsy though they debated the merits of disclosure. Service provider 4, a social service worker, supported the view that disclosure was a personal choice but, for those having seizures at work, that choice was not available. Service provider 5 was equally ambivalent, saying that given the stigma of epilepsy as a disability and chronic medical condition, people should not be forced to disclose, adding we also have 'to protect my interests as a person with the condition'. Among other service providers, there was consensus that disclosure was a personal choice.

While service providers said little about individual resilience, their views reinforced the fact that people with epilepsy faced extremely challenging employment situations and that services to reduce such disadvantage were limited. They seemed to agree that people with epilepsy, who succeeded against all odds, had an extra attribute, 'force' or 'God's grace' not available in others, to use the words of Service provider 5.

Implications

Despite the barriers encountered in their journey towards gaining and maintaining employment, despite the odds stacked against them, the findings showed that participants had demonstrated remarkable resilience by overcoming chronic unemployment. Employment barriers faced aligned with those reported previously (Dewa et al., 2014; Sebit & Mielke, 2005). Delayed medical treatment compromised education and vocational training—key factors for acquiring skills and for positive employment outcomes. As pointed out by service providers, in the absence of reliable public services, people with epilepsy were left to self-manage their adversity. Faced with adversity, participants used their individual resilience. Previous studies reached the same conclusion (Day, 2008; Ring et al., 2016; Taylor et al., 2011; Edward et al., 2015).

Resilient individuals acquired skills needed for jobs, despite the odds stacked against them. Findings showed that resilient individuals had skills and some were training to acquire more. The findings showed that skills were important if people with epilepsy were to have favourable employment outcomes. Service providers supported this view, pointing out that people with epilepsy lacked the skills required for employment. Those who acquired skills walked an extra mile, and showed resilience.

Resilient individuals achieved in the workplace beyond expectations. Previous research in Zimbabwe showed that people with epilepsy did not perceive their cognitive impairment to interfere with their functioning and work performance (Mugumbate & Nyanguru, 2013). This could be true given that participants in this research were able to work effectively. Workplace challenges emanated from incorrect knowledge about epilepsy, a situation found to be prevalent in Zimbabwe in previous studies (Mugumbate & Mushonga, 2013; Vyas, Wong, Yang, Thistle, & Lee, 2016). Prior studies showed negative attitudes among educated people (Mielke, Adamolekun, Ball, & Mundanda, 1997). A similar finding was reached in this study. Educated managers had incorrect knowledge of epilepsy, making the situation extremely challenging for workers with epilepsy.

Resilient individuals in this study had good seizure control and had a mastery of epilepsy. Previous studies reached the same conclusion (Ring et al., 2016; Taylor et al., 2011). As reported in other studies (Sebit & Mielke, 2005), health services were erratic and acted as a barrier to the employment chances of people with epilepsy. Resilient individuals were able to achieve greater control of seizures, perhaps because of the control they developed over their epilepsy. They were cognisant of side effects of medication and were able to control them effectively.

The findings of this research supported the argument that resilient individuals depended on their individual self-management abilities and environmental support systems (Ring et al., 2016). This study confirmed the role of social support systems in building resilience (Ring et al., 2016). An important support system for participants was the ESF. Service providers supported this view. Participants were members of the ESF who had benefitted from its medical and psychosocial interventions and often participated in support groups and advocacy work. This presented participants with an opportunity to manage their epilepsy and build the self-confidence to challenge negative attitudes. No doubt this was a factor that fostered their resilience. As members, they often interacted with service providers and other people in their situation. As one service provider said, their role was to misinform people with epilepsy of the notion that they had no potential. Further, the service providers advocated for opportunities for their members, and some members were exposed to employers who worked with the ESF.

Participants in this study showed that, despite the barriers to employment, they were able to overcome and achieve a better quality of life. This supports a view held by advocates of the resiliency model that, after disruption, resilient individuals are able to reintegrate in a manner that improves their quality of life and reduces their vulnerability (Richardson, 2002; Ring et al., 2016; Saburi, 2011). They bounce back. However, resilience alone was not enough, such factors as the economy and availability of services also impacted on employment opportunities.

Although the equal number of males and females did not necessarily mean that resilience was experienced equally between males and females in this study, the figures point in that direction. In this study, there were no noticeable differences between males and females regarding resilience. Service providers said women faced a 'triple burden' and, in light of this, their resilience was remarkable.

Inevitably, the research presented in this chapter had some limitations. First, it did not focus strongly on individual factors, such as vulnerability, personality, seizure type, treatment, or depression, as highlighted in previous studies (Day, 2008; Taylor et al., 2011). The research focused mainly on structural factors. Secondly, experiences of vulnerability were not explored, and participants were not always resilient. Despite these limitations, the study's conclusions have important implications for epilepsy work.

Vulnerability

Faced with numerous social challenges, most participants were vulnerable. Even those who were resilient had moments of vulnerability. Others had lost the confidence needed for job seeking and had given up looking for work. Yet others had psychological challenges. Mucha had become withdrawn in the workplace; Lameck had changed jobs; Rugare had worked harder; and Tindo, though she had worked hard, had stopped work, opting for self-employment, while Ashley and Tino kept on fighting. Munya and Saru had become suicidal. Mucha recounted that, initially, he had become 'very stressed' following his retrenchment. He had gone 'into a huge depression' and had withdrawn from friends, who had disassociated from him, leading to his social isolation. Some people had teased him, saying he was sick because his 'father had evil spirits or *chikwambo* [goblin]'. Mucha explained: 'I became a drunkard. I would go to the bar after school and get drunk. So that the community, when they say "things" [like I was possessed], I would not mind'. Saru, too, had contemplated suicide due to her social isolation: 'I had come to a situation where I even prayed behind my house that God should end my life'.

Conclusion

Despite the barriers encountered in their journey towards gaining and maintaining employment, the eight people with epilepsy reported in this study, who demonstrated tremendous individual resilience, showed how this enabled them to overcome some of the barriers they had encountered. They exhibited a strong 'fighting spirit' in seemingly hopeless situations and ongoing shame associated with their condition. The research concluded that, where employment support services were weak to address employment barriers, as in Zimbabwe, individual resilience acted as a strong coping mechanism that resulted in better employment outcomes for many. These findings have implications for policy and practice. Service providers in epilepsy work ought to add resilience building to their portfolio of strategies. Increasing people with epilepsy's knowledge and acceptance of their condition could be a starting point. However, this is only a coping mechanism that should not stop service providers and service users to advocate for government-provided employment services.

References

Day, K. (2008). *Quality of life: The role of psychological resilience*. Edinburgh: University of Edinburgh.

Dewa, E., January, J., Nyati-Jokomo, Z., Mafaune, P. T., Muteti, S., & Maradzika, J. (2014). Non-attendance of treatment review visits among epileptic patients in a rural district, Zimbabwe. *Journal of Public Health in Africa, 5*(2), 73–76.

Edward, K., Cook, M., & Giandinoto, J. (2015). An integrative review of the benefits of self-management interventions for adults with epilepsy. *Epilepsy & Behavior, 45*, 195–204.

Mielke, J., Adamolekun, B., Ball, D., & Mundanda, T. (1997). Knowledge and attitudes of teachers towards epilepsy in Zimbabwe. *Acta Neurologica Scandinavica, 96*(3), 133–137.

Mugumbate, J., & Mushonga, J. (2013). Myths, perceptions, and incorrect knowledge surrounding epilepsy in rural Zimbabwe: A study of the villagers in Buhera District. *Epilepsy & Behavior, 27*(1), 144–147.

Mugumbate, J., & Nyanguru, A. (2013). Measuring the challenges of people with epilepsy in Harare, Zimbabwe. *Neurology Asia, 18*(1), 29–33.

Munn, Z. (2008). Care delivery and self-management strategies for adults with epilepsy. *Journal of Advanced Nursing, 64*, 455–456.

Richardson, C. E. (2002). The metatheory of resilience and resiliency. *Journal of Clinical Psychology, 58*(3), 307–321.

Ring, A., Jacob, A., Baker, G., Marson, A., & Whitehead, M. (2016). Does the concept of resilience contribute to understanding good quality of life in the context of epilepsy? *Epilepsy & Behavior, 56*, 153–164.

Saburi, G. (2011). Stressors of caregivers of school-age children with epilepsy and use of community resources. *Neuroscience Nursing, 43*(3), 1–12.

Sebit, M. B., & Mielke, J. (2005). Epilepsy in sub-Saharan Africa: Its socio-demography, aetiology, diagnosis and EEG characteristics in Harare, Zimbabwe. *East African Medical Journal, 82*(3), 128–137.

Taylor, J., Jacob, A., Baker, G., Marson, A., Ring, A., & Whitehead, M. (2011). Factors predictive of resilience and vulnerability in new-onset epilepsy. *Epilepsia, 52*(3), 610–618.

Vyas, M. V., Wong, A., Yang, J. M., Thistle, P., & Lee, L. (2016). The spectrum of neurological presentations in an outpatient clinic of rural Zimbabwe. *Journal of the Neurological Sciences, 362*, 263–265.

World Health Organisation (WHO). (2016). Epilepsy. Retrieved October 16, 2016 from https://www.who.int/mediacentre/factsheets/fs999/en/

12 The integrative model for managing epilepsy (IMME)

The objective of this book is to increase the understanding of, and interventions to improve the quality of life of people with epilepsy in resource-limited settings; increase the understanding of, and interventions to reduce the income gap in epilepsy in resource-limited settings; increase the understanding of, and interventions to reduce the policy gap in epilepsy in resource-limited settings, and enhance the skills of those providing social interventions to improve the quality of life of people with epilepsy in epilepsy in resource-limited settings. This chapter brings these objectives strongly together to create a model for managing epilepsy. This won't be the first model. This chapter will start by giving an overview of information presented in previous chapters, then, this chapter will turn to a proposed integrative model of managing epilepsy (IMME), which is an improvement of the comprehensive epilepsy management model (CEMM).

Overview

Information box 12.1　Overview of epilepsy

Key perspectives

1　Spiritual perspective
2　Biological perspective

Key debates

1　Where does epilepsy come from (causes)?
2　How should epilepsy be stopped (treatment)?
3　What makes epilepsy more or few, easy or worse (determinants)?
4　What should be the position of people with epilepsy in society (status and recognition)?

DOI: 10.4324/9781003602866-12

Common understandings

1   Epilepsy reduces social approval.
2   It causes unexpected body movements, unconsciously.
3   It results in uncontrolled movements.
4   It impacts cognition.
5   It can't be fully explained or treated physically.
6   It is recurring but is not permanent.

Interventions

1   Medical
2   Psychosocial
3   Social
4   Economic
5   Human rights
6   Affirmation
7   Family/carer

Key determinants

1   Environment
2   Culture
3   Religion
4   Health system
5   Genetics
6   Income
7   Education
8   Policies
9   Comorbidities

Holistic and integrative health model

This model uses both traditional and modern medical approaches. The WHO and many countries support this idea, recognising that to achieve complete health coverage, all types of treatments should be included. Modern health systems should combine different methods to provide full and effective care. The model values the wisdom of traditional practices alongside the advancements of contemporary medicine, ensuring a more comprehensive and personalised approach to health. This integration helps bridge gaps in healthcare, making it more accessible and responsive to different cultural and medical perspectives. In the context of epilepsy, the holistic and integrative health model can be particularly beneficial. Alongside conventional treatments such as medication and surgery, incorporating complementary therapies like acupuncture, *panchakarma*, diet management, mindfulness practices and spiritual support can offer additional benefits. Acupuncture may help manage seizures and reduce medication side effects, while *panchakarma*, an ayurvedic detoxification process, can aid in balancing the body's energies. Mindfulness and spiritual practices can provide emotional and psychological support. This comprehensive approach not only helps manage symptoms more effectively but also addresses the overall well-being of individuals, improving their quality of life and offering a more rounded strategy for dealing with epilepsy.

The comprehensive epilepsy management model

In previous work, Mugumbate (2017) proposed a model for managing epilepsy grounded in Fraser's social justice approach. This model focuses more on social justice from an economic, cultural and political perspective.

Tools and models 12.1   Comprehensive epilepsy management model epilepsy

Key aspects	*Barriers to participation*	*Main requirements*
Economic redistribution	Medical	Adequate supply of free drugs and epilepsy management services.
	Misunderstanding	Adequate health education and promotion through publicity about the availability of treatment.
	Resources/funds	Policies to ensure funding is guaranteed.
	Lack of income	Accessible employment services and opportunities and social welfare support.
Cultural recognition	Beliefs	Educate employers, educators and stakeholders in employment about epilepsy. Provision of accurate information about epilepsy to change how culture represents epilepsy.
	Traditional treatments	Regulation and improvement of traditional treatments.
	Status recognition	Recognise the disabling nature of epilepsy and that people with epilepsy form a disadvantaged group especially women, workers and rural people with epilepsy. Targeted epilepsy antistigma and antidiscrimination legislation.
Political representation	Policy	Targeted national epilepsy legislation and management plans, for example, employment policy, disability policy and health policy. Domestication of regional and international instruments.
	Self-representation	Self-representation through support growth organisations and initiatives supporting people with epilepsy to build their sense of self. Ensure representation in all sectors including workplace boards, education boards.
	Justice	Easy access to courts. Clear formal processes to challenge injustice.

The model emphasises the economic, cultural and political aspects of epilepsy. The model could be used by service providers and people with epilepsy as a tool to plan or evaluate epilepsy programmes. Programmes that recognise that challenges facing people with epilepsy are economic, sociocultural and political in nature are likely to address the key challenges faced by people with epilepsy. Key aspects of the model are economic redistribution, cultural recognition and political representation. The key aspects are broken down into barriers, and requirements to address these barriers. The barriers encompass income, medical aspects, misunderstanding, policy, participation and justice. The model acknowledges the key role of biomedical treatment in the control of seizures but emphasises that ending seizures cannot be the end of managing the condition, there is a need for economic support to ensure access to medicines, and social support to ensure that the stigma of having epilepsy does not affect full participation in society.

If the main requirements for the success of this model were not available, this would result in structural inequality, described by Fraser as maldistribution, misrecognition and misrepresentation. Therefore, social justice is not achievable in the absence of any of the key aspects. The economic aspect ensures what Fraser termed economic restructuring, income transfer and labour reorganisation. The second aspect, cultural component, ensures revaluing of an epilepsy identity and building of sense of self (Fraser, 2010). The last component, the political, ensures the needs and claims of people with epilepsy are articulated. In between the aspects and requirements lay barriers to participation. Recalling that Fraser (2010) put parity of participation at the centre of economic, cultural and political justice, social justice would allow people with epilepsy to participate in society as peers. To achieve participation, the model recognises some aspects that should be streamlined, such as gender, age geographical location, seizure type and research needs. Mainstreaming is required to ensure that children, the elderly services, rural dwellers, women and those with absence seizures are not left out of epilepsy programmes.

Therefore, it is suggested that the results could be generalised to most African countries because the issues reported herein represent an Africa-wide challenge in managing epilepsy (Birbeck, 2000; Duggan, 2013; Mushi et al., 2011; Nuhu, Fawole, Babalola, Ayilara, & Sulaiman, 2010). Literature showed that epilepsy stigma existed in Indigenous, Muslim and Christian African societies, and in urban and rural areas (Birbeck, 2000; Mushi et al., 2011). Like Zimbabwe, most African communities have limited public services offering healthcare, social welfare and employment support (International Labour Organisation [ILO], 2015, 2016; World Health Organisation [WHO], 2005, 2011, 2015, 2016). Although this study focused on epilepsy in Zimbabwe, the findings may well have a strong bearing on epilepsy and disability in Africa. Therefore, the model suggested in the next section has been designed with the African situation in mind.

However, there are some shortcomings with this model, the main one being that it ignores the different perspectives on epilepsy. Further, the model puts participation at the centre. While this is important, and addresses the challenge of empowerment, the approach relegates systems in which people with epilepsy live to the periphery and does not fully recognise capability. From an Ubuntu perspective, the family, community, society, environment and spirituality are al_ systems that work together to provide people with epilepsy an opportunity to realise their potential (Mugumbate & Nyanguru, 2013a, 2013b), that is capability in the theory of Sen (Sen, 1997, 1985, 1999). In that regard, an improved model is being proposed.

Integrative epilepsy management model

This new model is an improvement of previous models. It is holistic, integrative, preventive, health system-centred, family-centred and multidisciplinary in orientation. With this new model, culture is seen as part of philosophy, capabilities are introduced and prevention is emphasised. It borrows from the author's previous work (Mugumbate, 2010; Mugumbate & Nyanguru, 2013a, 2013b, Mugumbate & Mushonga, 2013; Mugumbate & Gray, 2016, 2017a, 2017b, 2021; Mugumbate, Riphagenn, & Gathara, 2017; Mugumbate & Zimba, 2018; Mugumbate et al., 2022, 2023) and from WHO resources on epilepsy (WHO, 2022, 2024), including the intersectoral plan on epilepsy running from 2022 to 2031.

Tools and models 12.2   Integrative model of managing epilepsy

Key aspects	Barriers to capability and participation	Main requirements
Prevention	No focus on prevention	Improved public health and primary health services
Capabilities	Stigma	Education (schooling) Awareness of the condition
Economic recognition	Medical costs	Adequate supply of free drugs and epilepsy management services
	Misunderstanding	Adequate health education and promotion through publicity about the availability of treatment
	Resources/funds	Policies to ensure funding is guaranteed
	Lack of income	Accessible employment services and opportunities and social welfare support
Philosophical recognition	Non-recognition of other ways of knowing or perspectives	Learning from all philosophies
	Beliefs	Educate employers, educators and stakeholders in employment about epilepsy. Provision of accurate information about epilepsy to change how culture represents epilepsy
	Herbal treatments	Regulation and improvement of herbal treatments

Key aspects	Barriers to capability and participation	Main requirements
	Status recognition	Recognise the disabling nature of epilepsy and that people with epilepsy form a disadvantaged group especially women, workers and rural people with epilepsy. Targeted epilepsy antistigma and antidiscrimination legislation
Intersectoral response	No national epilepsy programme	A national epilepsy programme led by the government through the public health delivery system
Family and community centredness	More focus on the individual leaving the family and community	Opportunities for the family to contribute to health plans and opportunities for the community to contribute to prevention and mobilisation
Political recognition	Policy	Targeted national epilepsy legislation and management plans, for example, employment policy, disability policy, health policy. Domestication of regional and international instruments
	Self-representation	Self-representation through support growth organisations and initiatives supporting people with epilepsy to build their sense of self. Ensure representation in all sectors including workplace boards, education boards
	Justice	Easy access to courts. Clear formal processes to challenge injustice

Now that the IMME model has been provided, it is also important to provide a tool to assess the state of social issues when managing epilepsy in any given community or country. The tool proposed below takes a strengths and participatory approach. It requires people with epilepsy and carers to be involved in the assessment. Each assessor gives a rating of 1–3. Four assessors are required, including at least one from government and one from people with epilepsy. Two other assessors can come from non-government organisations, government, carer or health or disability entity. If an aspect is being fully prioritised or supported in the community or country, a rating of 1 is given. If average 0.5 or ½ is given. If not a priority, a 0 is given. A total score of 4 per aspect means fully prioritised while 0 means not prioritised. A score of over 21 per community or country means social issues are being prioritised, 14–20 means average, 7–13 means below average and 0–7 means there is no priority for social issues.

<table>
<tr><td colspan="6">Tools and models 12.3   IMME tool for assessing prioritisation of social issues</td></tr>
<tr><td>Key aspects priority</td><td>Assessor 1</td><td>Assessor 2</td><td>Assessor 3</td><td>Assessor 4</td><td>Rating</td></tr>
<tr><td>1 Prevention
2 Capabilities
3 Economic recognition
4 Philosophical
   recognition
5 Intersectoral response
6 Family and community
   centredness
7 Political recognition</td><td></td><td></td><td></td><td></td><td></td></tr>
<tr><td></td><td>/7</td><td>/7</td><td>/7</td><td>/7</td><td>/28</td></tr>
</table>

This tool provides opportunities for discussion. For example, each assessor will talk about their rating, focusing on the gaps and strengths that they see. If there are larger differences, then more discussion will be required.

Closing the gaps: the future of epilepsy management

The suggested will work and become sustainable if the role of families and communities are valued in the management of epilepsy, and the government creates, adopts and funds a national programme on epilepsy that acknowledges the role of local researchers and advocates, health, integrative health and allied health professionals, including social workers. Families play a crucial part in supporting individuals with epilepsy by providing care, managing medication and offering emotional support. Communities can offer additional layers of assistance, such as raising awareness, reducing stigma and facilitating access to resources. Involving these key stakeholders, the management of epilepsy can be more holistic and inclusive, addressing not only the medical but also the social and emotional aspects of the condition.

For these strategies to be effective, governments need to create, adopt and fund a national programme on epilepsy. This programme should recognise and incorporate the contributions of local researchers and advocates, who bring valuable insights and expertise to the table. By investing in such a programme, governments can ensure that the needs of individuals with epilepsy are met through a coordinated approach that includes research, public education and policy development. Adequate funding is essential to support research initiatives, develop educational resources and implement effective treatment and support services.

The role of health professionals, including integrative and allied health professionals such as social workers, is also vital. These professionals can provide comprehensive care that addresses various aspects of epilepsy management, from medical treatment to psychological support and social services. Integrating their expertise into the national programme ensures a multidisciplinary approach that can improve outcomes for individuals with epilepsy. Collaboration among these diverse professionals, the programme can offer more tailored and effective support, leading to better management and quality of life for those affected by epilepsy.

References

Birbeck, G. L. (2000). Seizures in rural Zambia. *Epilepsia, 41*(3), 277–281.

Duggan, M. B. (2013). Epilepsy and its effects on children and families in rural Uganda. *African Health Sciences, 13*(3), 613–623. doi:10.4314/ahs.v13i3.14

Fraser, N. (2010). *Scales of justice: Reimagining political space in a globalising world.* New York: Columbia University Press.

International Labour Organisation (ILO). (2015). *Disability inclusion strategy and action plan 2014–17.* Retrieved October 1, 2016 from https://www.ilo.org/global/topics/disability-and-work/WCMS_475650/lang–en/index.htm

International Labour Organisation (ILO). (2016). *Decent work and the 2030 Agenda for sustainable development.* Retrieved October 13, 2016. from https://www.ilo.org/global/topics/sdg-2030/lang–en/index.htm

Mugumbate, J., & Gray, M. (2016). Social justice and disability policy in Southern Africa. *Journal of Social Development in Africa, 31*(2), 7–24.

Mugumbate, J., & Gray, M. (2017a). Competing traditional and medical treatments of epilepsy in Harare, Zimbabwe. *African and Middle East Journal of Epilepsy* (accepted for publication).

Mugumbate, J., & Gray, M. (2017b). Individual resilience as a strategy to counter employment barriers for people with epilepsy in Zimbabwe. *Epilepsy and Behaviour.* March, 74C, 154–160. doi:10.1016/j.yebeh.2017.06.018

Mugumbate, J., & Gray, M. (2021). Employment rights for people with epilepsy in Zimbabwe: A social justice perspective. In V. Sewpaul, L. Kreitzer, & T. Raniga (Eds.), *The tensions between culture and human rights. Emancipatory social work and Afrocentricity in a Global World* (pp. 88–99). Calgary: University of Calgary Press.

Mugumbate, J., & Mushonga, J. (2013). Myths, perceptions, and incorrect knowledge surrounding epilepsy in rural Zimbabwe: A study of the villagers in Buhera District. *Epilepsy & Behavior, 27*(1), 144–147. doi:10.1016/j.yebeh.2012.12.036

Mugumbate, J., & Nyanguru, A. (2013a). Exploring African philosophy: The value of Ubuntu in Social Work. *African Journal of Social Work, 3*(1), 82–100.

Mugumbate, J., & Nyanguru, A. (2013b). Measuring the challenges of people with epilepsy in Harare, Zimbabwe. *Neurology Asia, 18*(1), 29–33.

Mugumbate, J., Riphagenn, H., & Gathara, R. (2017). The role of social workers in the social management of epilepsy in Africa. In M. Gray (Ed.), *The handbook of social work and social development in Africa* (pp. 168–180). London: Routledge.

Mugumbate, J., & Zimba, A. (2018). Epilepsy in Africa: Past, present, and future. *Epilepsy & Behavior, 7*, 239 – 241. doi:10.1016/j.yebeh.2017.10.009

Mugumbate, J. R. (2010). *Global Campaign Against Epilepsy (GCAE) Zimbabwe Report.* Epilepsy Support Foundation.

Mugumbate, J. R., Kissani, N., Acevedo, K., Mugumbate, C., Janneh, A., Lilia Núñez-Orozco, L., Mauricio, O. A., & Ibrahim, E. A. A. (2022). First aid (FA) and first guidance (FG) for epilepsy seizures: Key considerations and recommendations for developing regions of the world. *Journal of Social Issues in Non-Communicable Conditions & Disability, 1*(1), 11–24.

Mugumbate, R. (2017). Disability, employment, and social justice. Employment experiences of people with epilepsy in Harare, Zimbabwe. Doctor of Philosophy thesis. University of Newcastle.

Mugumbate, R., Klevor, R., Aguirre, M. O., Massi, G.D., Yaqoob, N., Acevedo, K., Yewnetu, E., Kanyabutembo, C., Ibrahim, E. A. A., Boutadghart, S., Janneh, A., & Kissani, N. (2023). Epilepsy awareness days, weeks, and months: Their roles in the fight against epilepsy and the intersectoral global action plan on epilepsy and other neurological disorders, *Epilepsy & Behavior, 148*, 109457, doi:10.1016/j.yebeh.2023.109457

Mushi, D., Hunter, E., Mtuya, C., Mshana, G., Aris, E. & Walker, R. (2011). Social-cultural aspects of epilepsy in Kilimanjaro Region, Tanzania: Knowledge and experience among patients and carers. *Epilepsy and Behaviour, 20*, 338–343.

Nuhu, F. T., Fawole, J. O., Babalola, O. J., Ayilara, O. O., & Sulaiman, Z. T. (2010). Social consequences of epilepsy: A study of 231 Nigerian patients. *Annals of African Medicine, 9*(3), 170–175. doi:10.4103/1596-3519.68360

Sen, A. (1985). *Commodities and capabilities.* London: Oxford University Press.

Sen, A. (1997). *On economic inequality* (2nd ed.). Oxford: Oxford University Press.

Sen, A. (1999). *Development as freedom.* Oxford: Oxford University Press.

World Health Organisation (WHO). (2005). *Atlas: Epilepsy care in the world.* Geneva: WHO.

World Health Organisation (WHO). (2011). *World report on disability.* Retrieved August 13, 2014 from https://www.who.int/disabilities/world_report/2011/en/

World Health Organisation (WHO). (2015). *Sixty-Eighth World Health Assembly adopts resolution on epilepsy.* Geneva: WHO.

World Health Organisation (WHO). (2016). *Epilepsy.* Retrieved October 16, 2016. from https://www.who.int/mediacentre/factsheets/fs999/en/

World Health Organisation (WHO). (2022). *Intersectoral global action plan on epilepsy and other neurological disorders 2022–2031.* Retrieved November 3, 2022 from https://www.who.int/news/item/28-04-2022-draft-intersectoral-global-action-plan-on-epilepsy-and-other-neurological-disorders-2022-2031

World Health Organisation (WHO). (2024). *Epilepsy.* Retrieved from https://www.who.int/news-room/fact-sheets/detail/epilepsy

Glossary

Advocacy Activities aimed at influencing public policy and resource allocation for specific issues, including health conditions like epilepsy.

Biological Pertaining to living organisms and the physiological processes that occur within them, often related to genetics and health.

Brain health A state of well-being in which the brain functions optimally, encompassing cognitive, emotional and social abilities, and the capacity to adapt to challenges.

Buen vivir Based on the philosophies of Indigenous people of Latin America, buen vivir means 'a good living.' It emphasises a holistic view of life where well-being, community and harmony with nature are priorities, advocating for equitable distribution of resources and respect for cultural diversity.

Capabilities Focuses on ensuring people have real opportunities to lead fulfilling lives. According to Sen (1985), social justice should be assessed by looking at the genuine opportunities people have to achieve well-being and lead fulfilling lives, rather than just their income or wealth.

Community work Efforts aimed at improving community well-being and development through collective action and participation.

Community-based interventions Programmes or strategies designed to improve health outcomes at the community level.

Confucianism Emphasises moral integrity, social harmony and the importance of relationships, advocating for a just society through the cultivation of virtue and proper roles within the family and community.

Counselling A professional relationship that helps individuals understand and address personal issues, emotions and behaviours through guided conversation and support. It includes the medium to long-term support and interventions required to empower a person with epilepsy. A key aspect of counselling is referring, which links individuals to relevant services, and it can be offered by experienced individuals or professionals.

Cultural attitudes Social norms and beliefs that influence perceptions and treatment of conditions like epilepsy.

Determinants Factors that influence an individual's or community's health and well-being, including social, economic, environmental and behavioural aspects.

Dharma The concept of duty or righteousness in Hinduism, Buddhism, Jainism and Sikhism, often associated with ethical living and fulfilling one's responsibilities in various aspects of life.

Discrimination Unjust or prejudicial treatment of individuals based on characteristics such as health status.

Employment The condition of having paid work or engaging in economic activities that provide income.

Epilepsy A neurological disorder characterised by recurrent seizures due to abnormal electrical activity in the brain. The noun epilepsy is derived from the Greek word *epilambanein*, meaning to be seized. The noun epilepsy can misrepresent the condition and contribute to stigma.

Epilepsy awareness Efforts aimed at increasing understanding and knowledge about epilepsy to reduce stigma and improve care.

Equity in health The principle of ensuring that everyone has fair access to health resources and services, regardless of their background.

Fafa Epilepsy in various African languages (e.g., kiSwahili [kifafa], isiNdebele [isifafa], isiZulu [sifafa] or chiShona [zvifaifa]).

First aid Immediate assistance is provided to someone who is injured or unwell, often until professional medical help arrives. It deals with medical emergencies posed by seizures and includes physical support and interventions to prevent injury and save lives.

First guidance Initial support or advice given to individuals seeking help or information, often in relation to health or social services. It is required to help the person understand what is happening, especially during a first seizure. First guidance deals with the information, social supports and interventions that are necessary when epilepsy starts and during or soon after a seizure has occurred.

Fquih An Islamic religious scholar.

Global North Countries typically characterised by higher income levels, advanced technology and greater political influence, often including Europe, North America and parts of Asia.

Global South Regions of the world are typically characterised by lower income levels and development, often including Africa, Latin America and parts of Asia.

Healthcare access The ease with which individuals can obtain needed medical services.

Human rights violations Breaches of the basic rights and freedoms to which all humans are entitled.

Human services Support services that improve the well-being of individuals and communities, including social work and healthcare.

Income The financial or material earnings received by individuals or households, often derived from employment, investments, or government assistance.

Integrated care A coordinated approach to healthcare that combines different services to improve patient outcomes.

Integrative   Referring to approaches that combine multiple methods or disciplines to create a comprehensive strategy for addressing complex issues, often enhancing overall effectiveness.

Interconnectedness   The concept that all individuals and communities are linked and that actions can have broader implications for the well-being of others.

International social work   The practice of social work that transcends national boundaries, focusing on global issues and the interconnectedness of societies.

Intersectoral global action plan (IGAP)   A framework developed by the WHO aimed at addressing gaps in knowledge, policy and treatment for epilepsy.

Jadu/dua   Witches in Afghanistan.

Jadugar   Magicians in Afghanistan.

Jinn   Evil spirits or demons in Arabic culture.

Karma   The principle in Hindu that actions have consequences, influencing an individual's future based on their deeds and behaviour.

Karuna   In Buddhism, the teaching focuses on suffering, its causes, and how to alleviate it mainly through compassion, non-discrimination and interconnectedness.

Livelihood   The means by which individuals secure the necessities of life, including work, income and resources.

Mortality and morbidity rates   Statistics that indicate the frequency of deaths and diseases in a population.

Noi-jeon-jeung   In Korea, the term for epilepsy was historically expressed as *gan-jil* (간질, 癎疾), which is derived from *dian-xian* (癲癇), meaning craziness or madness. In 2010/2011, the Korean Epilepsy Association and Korean Medical Association changed the terminology to *noi-jeon-jeung* (뇌전증), meaning 'cerebro-electric disorder.' This shift has also been adopted in Hong Kong, China and Japan.

Participation   The active involvement of individuals or communities in decision-making processes, programmes and policies that affect their lives.

Policy gaps   Areas where existing policies do not adequately address issues, particularly in healthcare and social services.

Prevention   Actions taken to reduce the risk of disease or injury, focusing on education, early detection and health promotion.

Primary healthcare   Basic healthcare provided at the community level, focusing on prevention, wellness and the treatment of common illnesses.

Quality of life   The general well-being of individuals, encompassing physical, mental and social aspects.

Quaternary healthcare   An extension of tertiary care that includes highly specialised and experimental treatments, typically provided in a limited number of centres with advanced technology.

Recognition   Acknowledgement and validation of diverse identities, cultures and experiences, particularly those of marginalised groups.

Redistribution   The reallocation of resources and opportunities to address inequalities and promote social justice.

Representation   The inclusion and visibility of diverse voices and perspectives in decision-making processes, policies and societal structures.

Resilience   The capacity of individuals or communities to recover from difficulties and adapt to challenges, particularly in the context of health and well-being.

Resource availability   The presence of financial, human and material resources necessary for effective healthcare.

Resource-limited settings   Environments where financial, human or material resources are insufficient to provide adequate services.

Sangoma   In African religion, a sangoma is a spiritualist, diviner, herbal healer and ritual specialist, also known as n'anga or nganga.

Secondary healthcare   Specialised medical services provided by specialists or hospitals after a primary care physician's referral, typically involving more complex diagnosis and treatment.

Seizure   A sudden, uncontrolled electrical disturbance in the brain that can cause changes in behaviour, movements, feelings or consciousness. The noun seizure can misrepresent the condition and contribute to stigma.

Seizure-related injuries   Injuries that occur as a result of seizures, including physical harm during convulsions.

Seva   In Hinduism and Buddhism, seva means selfless service performed for the benefit of others without expectation of reward or recognition.

Social casework   A method of social work focused on individual clients, addressing personal issues through assessment, intervention and support.

Social isolation   A state where individuals lack social connections and support systems.

Social justice   The concept of fair and just relations between individuals and society, focusing on issues like equality and rights.

Social policy   Guidelines and principles that govern how societal issues are addressed, particularly in areas like health, education and welfare.

Social work with groups   A branch of social work that focuses on facilitating group processes to address shared issues, promote social change and enhance well-being.

Spiritual   Relating to the non-physical aspects of life, often encompassing beliefs, values and practices that connect individuals to a higher purpose or meaning.

Status epilepticus   A medical emergency involving prolonged or repeated seizures that require immediate treatment.

Stigma   Social disapproval or discrimination against individuals based on characteristics such as having epilepsy.

Tertiary healthcare   Highly specialised medical care involving advanced procedures and treatments, usually provided in specialised facilities like major hospitals.

Ubuntu   An African philosophy, culture and religion, this concept conveys centredness on the community, justice, reciprocity and relations, conveying the idea that humans are human because of others, promoting solidarity and mutual obligation at individual, family, community, societal levels, environmental and spiritual levels.

Index

Note: **Bold** page numbers refer to tables.

For Product Safety Concerns and Information please contact our EU
representative GPSR@taylorandfrancis.com
Taylor & Francis Verlag GmbH, Kaufingerstraße 24, 80331 München, Germany